Herbal Remedies Bible: Life Saving And Healing Herbs For All Ailments

Easy Herbal Remedies For Over 100 Ailments

By: Arthur Bramble

TABLE OF CONTENTS

Publishers Notes

Disclaimer

This publication is intended to provide helpful and informative material. It is not intended to diagnose, treat, cure, or prevent any health problem or condition, nor is intended to replace the advice of a physician. No action should be taken solely on the contents of this book. Always consult your physician or qualified health-care professional on any matters regarding your health and before adopting any suggestions in this book or drawing inferences from it.

The author and publisher specifically disclaim all responsibility for any liability, loss or risk, personal or otherwise, which is incurred as a consequence, directly or indirectly, from the use or application of any contents of this book.

Any and all product names referenced within this book are the trademarks of their respective owners. None of these owners have sponsored, authorized, endorsed, or approved this book.

Always read all information provided by the manufacturers' product labels before using their products. The author and publisher are not responsible for claims made by manufacturers.

DEDICATION

I want to dedicate this book to Reina, she has been a complete inspiration to me while compiling this book, and to my readers; who's continual suggestions by way of reviews has helped me to implement their ideas for a better readers experience, keep them coming.

UNDERSTANDING WHAT HERBAL REMEDIES ARE

Herbal remedies use plant extracts or plants as a solution for health problems. This remedy can be prescribed by an herbalist, nutritionist or physician.

These remedies are often thought to be natural medicine or alternative medicine and are often referred to as herbal remedies as they do not need the prescription of a physician as they are not medication that is traditionally manufactured. The most typical form these remedies include poultices, oils, creams, tinctures and teas.

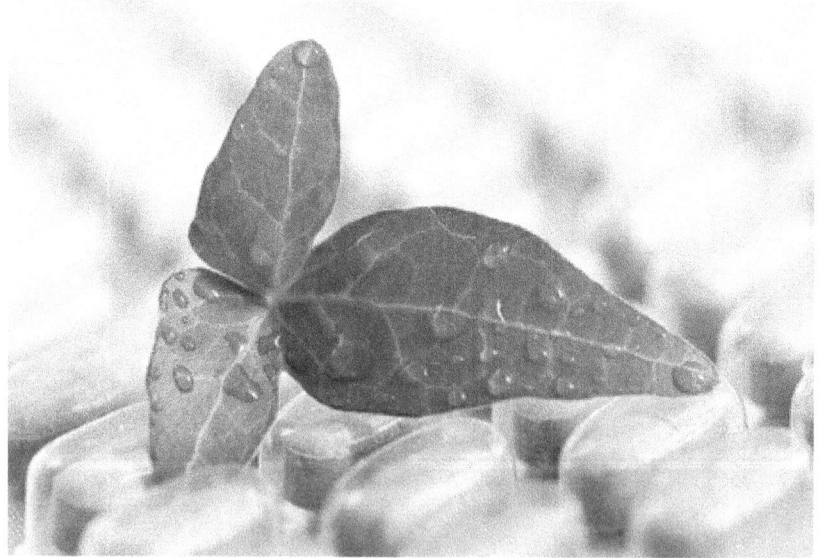

A lot of countries mandate that the herbalists have proper training and appropriate licensing before being able to prescribe any herbal remedies. In Europe, herbalists are plentiful and the pharmacies or apothecaries sell herbal remedies along with traditional medications. In countries like the United States herbal remedies tend to be sold in stores that sell vitamins and other similar supplements and not in the traditional pharmacies.

The formulas for herbal remedies are many and varied and a lot of these remedies have not been approved by the FDA (Food and Drug Administration) in the United States. Anytime an herbal remedy is being selected consumers ought to do their own research to find out about the listed ingredients and the benefits prior to making a purchase. If it is a case in which a pre existing illness is being treated by prescribed medications then care must be taken before an herbal remedy is taken as there can be contraindications when they are mixed.

The most popular way for a tea to be administered is in the form of a tea. The berries or leaves of the plant get crushed then are steeped in hot water for a few minutes to allow the nutrients and flavor of the plant to get into the water. These herbs can be sold loose or in tea bags.

The most common ones are green tea, rose hip and chamomile. With the loose leaves something known as a steeping ball is used. This steeping ball is made of metal has an outer covering of fine mesh which allows the flavor to get in the water and not leave any leaves behind when removed.

When it comes to a tincture for an herbal remedy it refers to an alcoholic extract which is most often prepared by mixing the berries and leaves of plants with ethanol. The leaves are soaked in the ethanol for a few days or even weeks to get the right concentration.

A popular tincture which is used as an antiseptic and used to treat cuts is a compound tincture of benzoin.

There are also topical remedies like poultices, oils and creams which are popular. The creams are usually a mix of salves and plant oil extracts which provide medicinal or cosmetic help. The covering for wounds is known as a poultice and is prepared by crushing the whole herb and not just the berries or leaves.

This mixture is placed right on the wound and then covered with a bandage. As a lot of herbs have soothing or antibacterial properties herbs have been utilized for many years to treat a number of injuries and illnesses.

BENEFITS OF HERBAL REMEDIES

Herbal medicine is a major part of alternative medicine. It is a great option for traditional medicine and can be used to treat and prevent a number of ailments. It is also known as medical herbalism, botanical medicine, herbalism and phytotherapy.

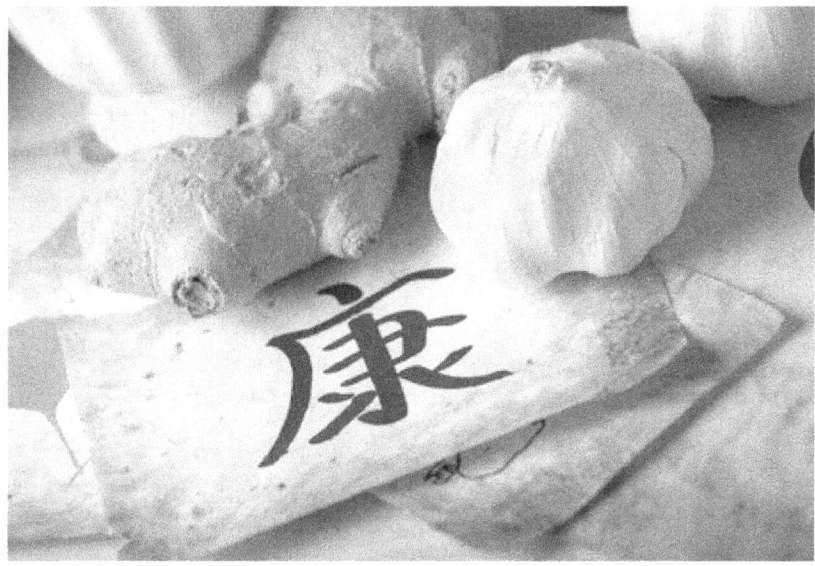

A simple structure of herbal medicine is made up of Western herbalism, Chinese herbalism and Ayurvedic herbalism. Quite a number of herbs are known for possessing superb medicinal properties. This type of medicine is one of the oldest types of medicine utilized for the treatment of psychological and physical ailments and also for the purpose of maintaining general health. This form of natural treatment has been practiced for many centuries to cure quite a number of illnesses. There are so many herbs out there that have great medicinal properties and can be used to prepare various medicines. A number of these herbs are extremely potent and do not have the lingering effects that the chemically made treatments do. The natural forms of treatment can be had as tablets, powdered or liquid extracts, ointments, essential oils or teas.

Benefits of Herbal Medicine

Health remedies and herbal medicines have a number of benefits, the most important being that it does not inhibit the natural healing process of the body. outlined below are a few of the advantages of opting for herbal options as forms of treatment to deal with ailments that can range from something as simple as the flu to something as chronic as cancer or diabetes.

Healing Naturally

As mentioned previously, herbal medicine does not affect the healing properties of the body. In contrast, these herbs actually boost the natural healing properties so that the process of recovery is much faster and the body can be in the best condition to promote that rapid healing. Quite a number of herbs work by triggering the glands to produce the necessary hormones. These hormones transport the signal of distress to the necessary areas to either inhibit or induce certain processes necessary for healing to take place.

Additional Benefits

Quite a few herbal remedies have specific instructions for use especially when it comes to exercise, rest and diet which enhance the way the herbs work by getting the body in such a state that it is much more receptive to treatment. Of course lifestyle and dietary changes can help in the long run to get the patient's body working well. When these alterations become routine and are maintained even after full recovery has been made, the chances of a recurrence of the same illness are significantly lowered.

Improved Immunity

Herbs do a lot for improving the immune system as they tend to boost the natural process of healing of the body and get rid of the bad things that cause illness. As a result, the body's natural defenses are strengthened against pathogens which trigger secondary or primary infections.

Nutrition and Metabolism

An improved metabolism is the result of a better lifestyle, a modified diet and a better immune system. In the long run this promotes improved absorption of necessary nutrients by the body. This is why more often than not the consumption of foods that are too oily or to fatty (junk food) are not recommended.

The consumption of caffeine and other stimulants is not recommended either. There are two reasons for this, junk food does not provide the body with the necessary variety or quantity of nourishment and the stimulants can inhibit the way medication should work. In a nutshell, inadequate nutrition affects the process of treatment and also affects the way the herbs work to help the body recover from whichever ailment.

Side-effects

Even though it would not be correct to state that allergies and side effects are nonexistent when it comes to natural treatments, it is factual that as the process of healing is more aligned with what nature had in mind, the side effects are much less when herbal medications are utilized and as long as they are taken as prescribed and the dosages are monitored by a professional herbalist, naturopath or any other individual that specializes in alternative methods of healing.

If the herbs are taken without supervision however, it can trigger side effects that can range from something as fatal as extreme toxicity or death to something that is no more that mild discomfort.

HERBAL REMEDIES A-H

ALOE VERA- This has long been used in folk medicine and when used externally it helps heal sores and burns and restores the tissues of the skin. It also helps with dandruff and blemishes and keeps the skin soft. It is strongest when used fresh and can also be ingested to help with stomach disorders and can also work as a laxative when dried.

Aloe is a succulent flowering plant that has a wide array of use, from soothing skin irritations to relieving constipation. Its scientific name is Aloe vera and has been known by other common names such as miracle plant, plant of immortality, Indian aloe, elephant's gall, and cape aloe.

Growing aloe

Aloe vera is a native of the African continent, specifically the southern and tropical regions of Africa including the islands off the coast of the continent and the Arabian Peninsula. It had been introduced to China and some parts of Europe in the 17th century. It has eventually been cultivated for its purportedly medicinal value. It needs about two to three years before it can be harvested for their juice. Cultivated aloe is harvested in early spring.

Aloe can grow on dry, loamy sand. It is propagated by roots that have been dug out from the parent plant. Another alternative way is to use rhizome cuttings after the aloe harvest and allowed to root before it can be transplanted. It is then spaced out at 31 inches in rows between rows. Approximately 5,000 aloes can be set per acre and takes about a year or two to mature.

Aloe vera appears as a circular clump of large, thick, and fleshy leaves directly from the roots as it has no stem. Its leaves coloured green to greyish green with mottled flecks of white. The leaves have small white teeth. When the flowers appear in summer, they come on a spike about three feet tall. Each yellow flower has appears singly and tubelike.

Benefits of aloe

Aside from its moisturising effect on the skin and its relieving effect on the constipated bowel, aloe has also benefited people with diabetes, asthma, and epilepsy. It has also been given to relieve fever, itching, and soreness. It has been applied externally for arthritis, burns, and psoriasis. People suffering from cold sores, frostbite, sunburn, and bedsores are believed to benefit from aloe application.

What to look out for

Topical application of aloe has no reported side effects. Prolonged use of aloe can cause hives and swollen, red eyelids. People with allergies to any member of the Lily Family, such as garlic, onions, tulips and the like, should not use this herbal remedy.

When taken internally, aloe can cause abdominal cramps and diarrhoea. Long term usage is often associated with kidney disorders, blood in the urine, low potassium levels, muscle weakness, weight loss, and heart problems. Loose bowel movements can decrease the absorption of most medications.

People with diabetes should check their blood glucose regularly as ingestion of aloe can drastically dip blood sugar levels. Those with blocked intestines such as Crohn's disease or ulcerative colitis should also steer clear. It can worsen haemorrhoids.

Aloe can also affect certain medications. People taking maintenance doses of digoxin should never take aloe as the latter lowers the electrolyte potassium, which can increase the toxic side effects of the drug. Blood thinning medications can also become more potent with aloe. Combining aloe with other stimulant laxatives such as bisacodyl, cascara, castor oil, senna, and the like as well as other diuretics, can dehydrate the body and cause electrolyte imbalance. Aloe can also affect herbs and other supplements. Potassium-lowering herbs such as licorice and horsetail may be dangerous. Phytoestroegens such as soy and herbal antivirals can also become affected.

Pregnant and breastfeeding women should never ingest aloe because there is risk of birth defects. Children should never be given aloe for ingestion.

How to use aloe

Historically, aloe has appeared to be used by ancient civilisations for a wide variety of conditions. It has been used as a versatile skin remedy and an effective laxative. The leaf is divided into two parts, the gel and the latex, which are used differently. The gel from aloe is jelly-like component of the inner leaves while the yellow latex lines the leaves' skin internally. It can be used on freckles.

When given for constipation, 100 to 200 milligrams of aloe may be taken in the evening. It takes about 10 hours for the herb to take effect. Alternatively, some people use 50 milligrams of aloe latex, but it might be unsafe. Liquid aloe extracts may be given at 30 millilitres every eight hours. The tincture of aloe is given at 15 to 60 drops when needed.

If used for psoriasis, a 0.5 per cent cream of aloe extract is applied every eight hours to remove plaques. It can also be applied three to five times daily when needed. The cream may also be given for genital herpes. Pure aloe gel may be applied on the surface of the skin for mild to moderate skin conditions.

Traditional uses for aloe involve inhaling its steam when set in a pan of boiling water for asthma or taking the gel with milk for people suffering from kidney problems.

Studies on aloe

Aloin, aloe-emodin, and barbaloin are strong laxative compounds found in aloes that had been classified by the US Food and Drug Administration (US FDA) as over-the-counter laxatives. In 2002, the US FDA removed laxative products that contain such ingredients because supplement manufacturers have failed to provide any data on safety. The sisterole content is being studied for its ability to slow down or stop inflammation.

Many initial studies have shown that topically applied aloe gel is beneficial for burns and abrasion. However, the gel cannot prevent burns from radiation therapy. A separate study has been able to show that aloes prevent or slow down the healing of wounds caused by deep surgery.

A two-year study by the National Toxicology program focused on the effect of ingesting whole leaf extract of aloe in rats. According to their data, the animals have developed tumours in their large intestines. More studies have to be done to relate this study to humans. Aside from this, separate studies have demonstrated that aloe will require increasing doses in order to have a laxative effect because the intestines become dependent on its stimulation.

References:

• Healthline. "What is Aloe? Dosing, Side Effects & More." 2010. http://www.healthline.com/natstandardcontent/aloe (accessed 30 Jun 2013).

• Mayo Clinic. "Aloe (Aloe vera) - MayoClinic.com." 2012. http://www.mayoclinic.com/health/aloe-vera/NS_patient-aloe (accessed 30 Jun 2013).

• Medline Plus. "Aloe: MedlinePlus Supplements." 2002. http://www.nlm.nih.gov/medlineplus/druginfo/natural/607.html (accessed 30 Jun 2013).

• RxList. "Aloe Effectiveness, Safety, and Drug Interactions on RxList." 2013. http://www.rxlist.com/aloe/supplements.htm (accessed 30 Jun 2013).

Health Library by iHerb. "Health Library - C573 - Aloe - Natural, Alternative - 21470." 2008. http://healthlibrary.epnet.com/GetContent.aspx?token=e0498803-7f62-4563-8d47-5fe33da65dd4&chunkiid=21470 (accessed 30 Jun 2013).

ANISE-   Anise is a flowering herb that grows in abundance in the eastern Mediterranean and Southwest Asia region. Its scientific name is Pimpinella anisum and is also called aniseed.

Anise aroma and taste has been compared to other comparable spices such as the star anise, liquorice, and fennel. It is also called hua hsian or sweet cumin.

Growing anise

Ancient Egyptians have cultivated anise for centuries. It is indigenous to Greece, Crete, and Asia Minor. It eventually spread to Rome and in the Middle Ages; Central Europe began cultivating the herb. The English have been growing this since the sixteenth century.

The anise plants grow from seeds which are sowed on loose but fertile soil, that is very well-drained. It should be near a warm shade and should be kept free from weeds. When planted in April, seeds will mature in autumn. Grown anise will have simple leaves near the base a bit pin like at the top. The flowers are white and eventually develop into an oval fruit called the aniseed.

Benefits of anise

Ancient Chinese medicine and Ayurvedic medicine in India have used anise for treatment to improve memory and to control excessive oiliness of the skin.

Anise has been used to treat menstrual cramps, to relieve gas, and to eliminate head lice and mites. It has also been used as a cough expectorant, a diuretic to increase urination and as an appetite stimulant. Some people use it to treat seizures, insomnia, relieve asthma, and to aid in nicotine addiction.

Women stand to benefit from anise' effect as a phytoestrogen, It can increase milk production during nursing, regulate flow of menstruation, help ease childbirth, provide relief from morning sickness, and increase libido. Men can also benefit from anise by using it to combat Andropause (male menopause).

Anise also has the ability to improve the absorption of iron from the diet. Its tea when used as a mouthwash can sweeten the breath and when swallowed can relieve sore throat.

What to look out for

Anise is generally safe, even for children, when taken in amounts similar to those in food. There is also no harmful effect when anise is applied on the scalp even if it is in combination with other herbs. It is safe for pregnant and breastfeeding women, although evidence has yet to be presented whether anise will cause harm in larger than usual amounts. Too much anise can trigger abortion in pregnant women.

Since anise is a phytoestrogen, conditions that react to spikes in oestrogen levels might worsen. People with cancers (breast, uterus, and ovary), endometriosis, and fibroids in their uterus should stay away from supplements that might contain anise or its active component, anethole.

Anise can lessen the effects of tamoxifen, oral contraceptives and oestrogen replacement hormone preparations. Tamoxifen is a drug used for controlling the amount of oestrogen in the body for people with oestrogen sensitive cancers.

Some people may develop allergies for anise when used on the skin, or when taken for conditions of the lungs and digestive tract. When the oil is ingested, it may cause pulmonary edema, seizures, and violent bouts of vomiting.

How to use anise

The greenish brown ribbed seeds from the fruit and the oil extracted from the seed are the most commonly used components of anise. Sometimes, its roots and leaves are also used as herbal medicine.

Anise has been used in Western cuisine to add flavour and aroma to food, refreshments, and sweets because of its similarity in taste with liquorice. However, most parts of Asia have been using anise and its similar tasting spice, star anise. Since 1999, anise has been replaced by this relatively cheaper spice, especially in the West. The seeds are used whole or powdered. Picarones, champurrado, and mustaceoe are some dishes that rely on anise for flavour.

Anise is given as tea to nursing women and to those experiencing painful menstruation. It is deemed possibly effective for menstrual pain. There is a product that contains anise, saffron, and celery seed which effectively lessens the gravity and duration of discomfort during the whole cycle. For the first three days of menstruation, take 500 milligram of this preparation every eight hours.

For dyspepsia, about 300 to 500 milligrams of the seed or 0.1 to 0.3 millilitres of the essential oil are usually given to provide relief. There are very few preparations that contain pure anise and there has yet to be a standard to set its dosage for clinical use. When mixed with a tablespoon of sugar, three drops of anise essential oil will relieve colic.

The essential oil may be given for inhalation to relieve congestion of phlegm in the windpipe, especially in asthma and productive coughing. Tea made from anise tea strained with honey and glycerine can be used for this purpose. It can also improve memory and helps clear the skin from excess oils.

Studies on anise

One of the major flavour components of anise is anethole that is also found in star anise (scientific name Illicium verum). This makes up 85 per cent of its essential oil. It also has estragole, gamma-hymachalen and methyl chavicol.

According to an Agricultural Research Service study published in 2008, anise is rich in phenylpropanoids. These compounds have shown significant effect against Plasmodium falciparum, a parasite that causes malaria in humans, and Mycobacterium intracellulare, the bacteria that triggers infections in patients with poor immune systems.

A 2012 study published in the Journal of Clinical Research and Healthcare Management evaluated the performance of aniseed against bacteria through an in vitro experiment. It has been able to prove that aniseed extract has a great potential against Pseudomonas, Staphylococcus, Klebsiella, Streptococcus, and Escherichia. The researchers have recommended it as an adjunct to standard antibiotics in order to lower the incidence of bacterial resistance.

Another study in 2012 funded by the Research Institute for Islamic and Complementary Medicine of Tehran University of Medical Science reviewed the medicinal benefits of anise. It has been able to prove the claims that folk medicine has attributed to anise being a natural antimicrobial and antioxidant.

References:

• AltMD. "Anise." 2008. http://www.altmd.com/Articles/Anise--Encyclopaedia-of-Alternative-Medicine (accessed 22 May 2013).

• Botanical.com. "Anise." 1995. http://botanical.com/botanical/mgmh/a/anise040.html (accessed 22 May 2013).

• Drugs.com. "Anise." 2009. http://www.drugs.com/npc/anise.html (accessed 22 May 2013).

• Herbs 2000. "Anise." 2002. http://www.herbs2000.com/herbs/herbs_anise.htm (accessed 22 May 2013).

• WebMD. "Anise." 2005. http://www.webmd.com/vitamins-supplements/ingredientmono-582-

@Arthur Bramble@

ANISE.aspx?activeIngredientId=582&activeIngredientName=ANISE (accessed 22 May 2013).

BASIL- Basil is a popular kitchen herb that is sometimes called sweet basil or Saint Joseph's wort. Its scientific name is Ocimum basilicum and is a relative of the mint family. The herb is indigenous to India but is often associated with traditional Italian and Thai cuisine. The term comes from the Greek word basileus which means "king." Some herbalists have associated it with the mythical creature, basilisk, because it is said to produce a lot of snakes when crushed with a big stone.

Growing basil

For five millennia, the tropical regions of Asia have cultivated basil and its various hybrids. The basil grown in Asia has a stronger flavour similar to clove compared to the ones grown in the Mediterranean.

Basil can be grown from cut stems which have been suspended in water for a fortnight or until its roots develop. Once the roots appeared, they can be planted indoors in a pot. Just make sure they're placed in the sunniest part of the room. If the stem produces flowers, they become woody and the amounts of essential oil produced in the leaves on that stem stops. These flowers eventually produce seed pods that can also be used for planting.

Benefits of basil

Basil oil is said to have antioxidant, antiviral, and antimicrobial effects. It also showed major potential for use as anti-cancer. There are compounds in the plant that helps in blood thinning. Flavonoids such as orientin and vicenin are present in basil and can protect the body at the cellular level.

As a folk remedy, basil has been used to treat convulsions, hearing impairment, gout, hiccups, impotence, insanity, and whooping cough.

Traditional Ayurvedic medicine has used basil as treatment for stress asthma and diabetes. It can relieve spasms of the digestive tract, promote appetite, treat oedema, and expel worms. Women consume basil before and after giving birth to improve their blood circulation and to increase milk production during nursing.

Nutrition wise, basil is rich in Vitamin A because of its abundant supply of beta-carotene. This powerful antioxidant improves cardiovascular health by protecting the lining of the blood vessels from free radicals and prevents it from oxidising cholesterol. When oxidised cholesterol is gone, there would be no build-up of atherosclerotic plaque thus lowering the risk for a heart attack or stroke. It is also rich in magnesium, an electrolyte that helps the muscles and blood vessels ease up. Once relaxed, blood flow improves and the risk for spasms or irregular heart rhythms goes down.

What to look out for

When used as food, basil is generally safe. However, some people report having their blood sugar drop when using basil as a herbal remedy. Using basil might be harmful as it contains estragole, a chemical that could trigger the development of liver cancer.

Basil is a popular produce and are readily available in the local grocer's. To get the most out of it, opt for the ones that are grown organically or those that are sourced within the area. Irradiation of imported basil may allow it to stay fresh during transit but it could greatly diminish the amount of nutrients you can get out of it.

How to use basil

As an herbal remedy, the whole herb is used. In the West, it is often gathered around July.

Asian cuisine has used basil in various dishes. It uses a wide variety, from sweet basil, Thai basil, lemon basil, or holy basil. It is often cooked fresh and added as one of the last ingredients. It can be kept for a week inside an airtight bag in the refrigerator. Other substances that may be found in basil include myrcene, pinene, ocimene, terpineol, and caryophyllene.

One of the most common Ayurvedic remedies for basil is to improve the function of the urinary system. Equal amounts of basil leaves and honey is said to reduce or eliminate the kidney stones present.

As a poultice or ingesting basil leaves are the means of relieving inflammation and pain. For those with arthritis, tooth ache, and muscle pain a poultice of heated leaves of basil is effective. It releases eugenol which prevents the substances which are produced by the body that causes swelling and pain. It can also be rubbed on bruises and wounds.

Herbalists would determine the dose of basil based on the patient's age, health, and condition. At present, there is no scientifically proven standard that provides the adequate dose for basil.

If possible, go for fresh basil over the dried variety. Aside from being more flavourful, the amount of essential oils and nutrients are still intact. Keep it wrapped in a damp towel inside the refrigerator to store. When frozen, keep it in air tight containers or in ice trays covered with stock. If fresh basil is not around, dried basil will do as long as you keep it in a tightly sealed container in a cool, dark, and dry place to make it last for half a year.

Studies on basil

Different types of basil can have a variety of smells because each variety can have a different mix of essential oils. Those that smell like cloves have a high proportion of eugenol. The lemony scent can be attributed to the presence of citral and limonene. Some hybrids that smell like camphor contain camphene while those that seem like liquorice are rich in anethole.

In 1989, there was a study that demonstrated the ability of basil oil to repel insects and to exert an antifungal effect. In the same year, the antimicrobial effects of basil were also studied and it has been used to treat infections of the urinary tract. This was further confirmed in another separate study a decade after. The constituents of basil oil are deadly to mosquitoes.

There is a 2005 study published in the Journal of Agricultural Food Chemistry which showed that treating basil seeds with 0.5 per cent of chitosan concentration can increase its growth and the amount of its phytochemicals between 17 to 21 per cent. Here's your chance to have a say in what future content is placed in this book.

References:

• Botanical.com. "A Modern Herbal | Basil, Bush." 1995. http://botanical.com/botanical/mgmh/b/basbus17.html (accessed 22 May 2013).

• Georgetown University Medical Center. "URBAN HERBS: Basil." 1989.

http://pharmacology.georgetown.edu/urbanherbs/Basil.htm (accessed 22 May 2013).

• LIVESTRONG.COM. "Medical Benefits of the Basil Herb." 2010. http://www.livestrong.com/article/248798-medical-benefits-of-the-basil-herb/ (accessed 22 May 2013).

• Webmd.com. "BASIL: Uses, Side Effects, Interactions and Warnings - WebMD." 2005. http://www.webmd.com/vitamins-supplements/ingredientmono-303-BASIL.aspx?activeIngredientId=303&activeIngredientName=BASIL (accessed 22 May 2013).

• World's Healthiest Foods. "WHFoods: Basil." 2003. http://www.whfoods.com/genpage.php?tname=foodspice&dbid=85 (accessed 22 May 2013).

BLACK COHOSH- Black cohosh or black snakeroot, fairy candle, or black bugbane is a Native American favourite herb. It has potential for use as a sedative and relief of pain. Current use for Actaea racemosa (or for some, Cimifuga racemosa) is for alleviating the symptoms of menopause, insomnia, and mood swings. This is a relatively safe herb to use for menopausal symptoms for up to six months, according to the American College of Obstetrics and Gynaecology.

Growing black cohosh

Black cohosh is an herbal medication that is found along the rich, shady woodlands of North America. It is a tall, flowering herb having attributes similar to the members of the buttercup family. It will grow in heavy and moist soil. It often grows in the wild. Cultivation of black cohosh may be through pollination of various insects that has been attracted to its fetid smell.

Benefits of black cohosh

Since 2002, the dangers of hormone replacement therapy have scared most pre-menopausal women to resort to herbal therapy with black cohosh. Although the evidence has yet to prove otherwise, it is still being marketed as such. It can also relieve painful menstruation and regulate it.

Approximately 45 per cent of nurses and midwives use black cohosh to induce labour. However, there aren't any credible scientific evidence for it to be recommended for use in most patients. It has also been used to slow down the progressive bone weakness that comes after menopause. Although it's use has lowered the risk for weak bones, there are no data that proves it can lower the incidence of fractures for post-menopausal women.

What to look out for

There is scientific evidence that has shown the absence of black cohosh' estrogenic effect. There is currently no study on the effects of long term use of the herb on humans. Experiments on mice for cancer are contradictory.

What is known is the liver damage it might cause when using black cohosh, according to anecdotal evidence. Although there is no conclusive evidence for such adverse effect, Australia's Therapeutic Goods Administration has required a warning label on any products containing black cohosh.

There are reported side effects when black cohosh is taken. Dizziness, headaches, sweating, intestinal upset, a drop in blood pressure and slow heartbeats have been reported. Experts have hypothesized that since the herb grows in the wild, there could have been some unintentional mix-up of other harmful plants. Side effects may also be seen in people who take very high doses of the herb.

To be on the safe side, women who are pregnant, diagnosed with oestrogen sensitive cancers or endometriosis, children under 18, those with a very high risk for liver disease, and those allergic to aspirin should avoid black cohosh. It has the ability to stimulate the female ovaries and makes them a potent herb when taken for any other indication other than for relieving hot flashes.

There are also some medications that might interact with black cohosh. Most of these drugs affect the liver, especially those that rely heavily on the latter to get eliminated or become activated by the body. Atorvastatin, cisplatin, amitriptyline, codeine, fentanyl, metoprolol, olanzapine, odansetron, tramadol, acetaminophen, isoniazid, methotrexate, phenytoin, and other similar medications are those that have to be used with precaution when taken together with black cohosh.

How to use black cohosh

The Native Americans have been using black cohosh mostly for conditions of the female reproductive system and for sore throat, depression, and kidney disorders. When European settlers came in, they continued the use of black cohosh, which was also called black snakeroot. People used to apply it directly on the skin to improve skin conditions such as warts, acne, and unwanted moles.

There are a variety of preparations that contain standard amounts of black cohosh. Tablets may contain 40 to 80 milligrams. Tinctures are rare, but when used every dose is about 2 to 4 millilitres dissolved in water every eight hours. Teas are more traditional formulation that will contain 20 grams of black cohosh per bag to be dissolved in 34 millilitres of water. It should be boiled until reduced to a third of its volume and strained before being stored. It should be consumed within 48 hours, given one cup of black cohosh tea thrice daily.

Germany has approved its use as therapy for painful symptoms associated with menstruation and for relieving menopausal symptoms. When black cohosh is used to relieve the discomforting effects of menopause, 20 to 80 milligram tablets of the extract are taken every 12 hours. A dose higher than 900 milligrams is dangerous. For osteoporosis in women past their menopause, it's given at 40 milligrams daily.

Studies on black cohosh

The primary active compound in black cohosh is its terpene glycoside plus actein and cimifugoside. Since it has been traditionally used for gynaecological conditions, black cohosh had been originally associated as a phytoestrogen. However, there were published studies from 2002 to 2009 that were able to disprove the presence of such. The data used on these studies were able to establish that it's the presence of methyserotonin that could activate serotonin receptors. A research published in 2007 was able to show that triterpene glycosides in black cohosh could stop bone loss caused by cytokines.

At present, black cohosh has been used mainly as the go to remedy for women's gynaecological conditions. Studies in 2005 and 2006 have cast some doubts on its potency, as the results are mostly dose dependent. In a 2007 study, researchers were able to isolate some compounds from black cohosh that might benefit osteoporosis. A recent 2011 study was able to show black cohosh' ability to relax the smooth muscles of the blood vessels which might be of use to people with hypertension.

There are preliminary studies being done on the effect of black cohosh on arthritis, especially when combined with other herbs such as willow, sarsaparilla, poplar, and guaiacum resin. Although there is potential for this combination, clinical trials on humans have yet to prove its usefulness.

References:

• American Family Physician. "Black Cohosh." 2003. http://www.aafp.org/afp/2003/0701/p114.html (accessed 23 May 2013).

- Health Library by iHerb. "Black Cohosh." 2006. http://healthlibrary.epnet.com/GetContent.aspx?token=e0498803-7f62-4563-8d47-5fe33da65dd4&chunkiid=21584 (accessed 23 May 2013).

- Memorial Sloan-Kettering Cancer Center. "Black Cohosh." 2007. http://www.mskcc.org/cancer-care/herb/black-cohosh (accessed 23 May 2013).

- University of Maryland Medical Center. "Black cohosh." 2011. http://www.umm.edu/altmed/articles/black-cohosh-000226.htm (accessed 23 May 2013).

WebMD. "Black Cohosh." 2009. http://www.webmd.com/vitamins-supplements/ingredientmono-857-black%20cohosh.aspx?activeIngredientId=857&activeIngredientName=black%20cohosh (accessed 23 May 2013).

BUCKTHORN- The common sea buckthorn is a spiny woody shrub that is found locally in the sea crags and fixed sandbanks of Eastern Europe and some parts of Asia. Its common names are finbar, purging thorn, sallow thorn and sea buckthorn. Its scientific name is Hippophae rhamnoides. It is often mistaken for another herbal medication, the wolfberry.

Growing buckthorn

The buckthorn is a thorny shrub that can grow from 7 to 13 feet high. Its leaves are narrow and spear-shaped with flowers that have no petals. It eventually grows into an oval or roundish fruits that grow in bunch of pale yellow to dark orange. This plant is found in Europe from Britain to Norway and as far away as Spain. In Asia, it is found in Japan and Himalayas. Countries such as Germany, France, Finland, India, and Nepal cultivate it commercially. At present, China is the largest producer of the plant, although it is originally from Nepal.

Buckthorn is planted as seedlings during spring. It also needs a lot of light as the plant dislikes being in the shade. Distances are often set at 3 to 6 metres between each other, which makes it about 1,900 saplings per 2.471 acres.

Benefits of buckthorn

Although small, the fruits of the buckthorn are very rich in ascorbic acid, more than what oranges and lemons can offer. As an herbal remedy, buckthorn fruits can protect cells from damage, better recovery from stress, regulate the immune system, and hasten tissue regeneration. It can also protect from liver damage, prevent plaque from forming easily in the blood vessels, and better resistance to infections. It can also improve eyesight and slow down the ravages of time.

The leaves and flowers are used for arthritis, ulcers in the digestive system, gout, and rashes on the skin brought about by measles. Teas made from buckthorn leaves supply vitamins, amino acids, fatty acids, and minerals. It can also improve blood pressure and lower bad cholesterol while boosting immunity.

The seed of the buckthorn can be made into oil which has a variety of uses as well. It can loosen phlegm in those suffering from asthma, relieve the pain from angina, preventing cardiovascular diseases caused by high cholesterol, and as an adjuvant for cancer therapy.

Some people use the buckthorn berries and seed oil on the skin to heal and prevent further damage from sunburn radiation. It also hastens wound healing in bedsores, burns, wounds, acne, dermatitis, and eczema. There are also claims that buckthorn can effectively treat stretchmarks caused by pregnancy.

What to look out for

When used as food, buckthorn is safe. Its content in jams, pies, drinks, and other dishes have enough buckthorn to provide nutrients. It has shown relative safety when used in clinical studies for up to three months. In clinical trials where buckthorn showed its potential as an herbal medication, about 5 to 45 grams of the seed oil and about 300 millilitres/one cup of buckthorn juice per day are used.

There is little evidence on the long term effects of buckthorn use on pregnant and nursing women. For people who will undergo surgery within a fortnight/2 weeks should stay away from buckthorn consumption as it can slow blood clotting. Avoid using this herb with other blood thinners such as aspirin, clopidogrel, enoxaparin, warfarin, and other related medications.

At present, there is no standard clinical dose for buckthorn. When used, the herbalist relies on the various factors that might affect its function in the body. Manufacturers often indicate how their products are going to be used so it's best to follow the labelled instructions or consult a healthcare professional.

How to use buckthorn

The fruits of the buckthorn are used in a lot of products. However, it is quite expensive as it takes about 6 to 8 years before it can be harvested with some difficulty.

It is used in France as a fruit juice or as one of the constituents of its mixed drinks. The berries are also used as fruit based wines or sweet jams. It is also made as a tea in India.

Buckthorn has been the miracle cure of many Asian countries, including China, India, and Pakistan. Buckthorn has been make use of in Tibetan and Ayurvedic systems of herbal therapy for more than a hundred centuries. The Chinese traditional medicine has employed the buckthorn for digestive ailments, respiratory irritations, and conditions that affect circulation. In Tajikistan Buckthorn flowers have been used as a skin softener. Extracts from the branches and the leaves are used to treat irritation of the intestines in Mongolia. Russians employ the oil and fruit for skin irritations. The oil extract is used for the eye conditions. Economically, buckthorn is used for cosmetics and to prevent soil erosion.

At present, there is inadequate clinical evidence for its claims in cardiovascular health, liver disease, as well as infections of the digestive tract, dry eye, and colds. Preliminary studies have shown its effectiveness for these conditions.

Studies on buckthorn

Buckthorn contains ascorbic acid, carotenoids, tocopherols, flavonoids, and lipids. The flavonoids in the leaves and fruits have antioxidant and anti-cancer properties as well as the tocopherols. The carotenoids are able to reduce the incidence of macular degeneration due to aging including added antioxidant potency to the mix.

In separate studies in 2001 and 2005, researchers have been able to show that extracts of buckthorn can effectively inhibit certain bacteria (Bacillus, Listeria, and Yersinia). Another study also showed buckthorn extracts preventing Heliobacter pylori from increasing which also collaborated with the data in 2002 which showed buckthorn's anti-ulcer activity in rats.

When researchers conducted clinical trials on the effect of buckthorn on the skin in 2000, there was no significant improvement in patients with dermatitis when seed and pulp oil of buckthorn were used for over four months. In the same year, another clinical trial was done to show its effects on the cardiovascular system. The researchers were able to prove that buckthorn berry oil can act as a blood thinner, although the mechanism involved is unclear.

References:

- Globinmed.com. "Hippophae rhamnoides." 2009. http://www.globinmed.com/index.php?option=com_content&view =article&id=83214:hippophae-rhamnoides&Itemid=146 (accessed 23 May 2013).

- LIVESTRONG. "The Benefits of Sea Buckthorn." 2011. http://www.livestrong.com/article/404532-the-benefits-of-sea-buckthorn/ (accessed 23 May 2013).

- NYU Langone Medical Center. "Sea Buckthorn." 2007. http://www.med.nyu.edu/content?ChunkIID=214734 (accessed 23 May 2013).

- WebMD. "Hippophae Rhamnoides (SEA BUCKTHORN)." 2009. http://www.webmd.com/vitamins-supplements/ingredientmono-765-Hippophae%20Rhamnoides%20(SEA%20BUCKTHORN).aspx?activ eIngredientId=765&activeIngredientName=Hippophae%20Rhamno ides%20(SEA%20BUCKTHORN) (accessed 23 May 2013).

- Drugs.com. "Sea Buckthorn." 2004. http://www.drugs.com/npp/sea-buckthorn.html (accessed 23 May 2013).

BURDOCK- Burdock is a plant whose edible roots are used by folk herbalists as a blood purifier and its seeds are valued for its memory enhancing and anticancer properties. Its scientific name is Arctium lappa and is known by other common names such as beggar's buttons, fox's clote, great burr, happy major, love leaves, and thorny burr. In other languages, burdock is referred to as rhubarb du diable, niu bang zi, and bardane geante. The term "arctus" comes from Greek which meant bear, insinuating the bear's rough fur while "lappa" comes from Celtic word that meant to seize.

Growing burdock

Burdock is a native of temperate regions. It grows well in soil rich in nitrogen and in disturbed plots. It can be seen on waste ground and in fairly damp areas. It is found in Scandinavia, the Mediterranean, British Isles, Russia, Middle East, and Asia. Poisonous belladonna and deadly nightshade resemble burdock roots so keep away from gathering wild burdock.

Freshly tilled soil rich in humus and exposed to sunlight are just the right conditions for growing burdock. It reacts immediately to nitrogen-based fertilisers. It is sown in midsummer using its seeds and harvested after three to four months in late autumn. Very seldom will people contemplate on cultivating burdock but those who want to harvest the roots grow them in good soil. About 1,500 to 2,000 pounds of dry roots per acre may be harvested.

Burdock is a very tall plant as it can grow up to nine feet. Its large, alternating, and heart-shaped leaves are attached on long stalks and have hairy undersides. Its purple flowers are grouped on globular flower heads which bloom in midsummer. The flower heads are surrounded by burrs while its long, flat brownish grey fruits are covered with short hairs and appear wrinkly and contain a single seed. Its roots are fleshy, wrinkled, and covered with soft, white hairy leaf stalks. Externally, the roots are greyish brown but has white flesh and covered with thick bark. It can grow up to three feet and more than an inch thick.

Benefits of burdock

Burdock is beneficial for promoting urine flow, lower fevers, and cleaning the blood from impurities. It has also been given to treat colds, some types of cancers, problems in the gastrointestinal tract, joint pains, bladder infections, and complications that may arise from syphilis. Some people have used it for managing hypertension, hardening of the arteries, liver conditions, and poor sex drive. When applied externally, it's given for dry skin, acne, psoriasis, and eczema.

What to look out for

As a food, burdock is very safe aside from being very rich in antioxidants. Very little is known if burdock is safe when taken in doses for herbal remedies. To be on the safe side, pregnant and breastfeeding women should not use burdock or any of its extracts.

Ulcers, irritable bowels, dehydration, electrolyte imbalance, or excessive stomach acids might get worse with burdock use. People with allergies to ragweed, chrysanthemums, marigolds, daisies, and other related flowers might become hypersensitive to burdock.

When applied on the skin, burdock might cause some allergies. People with scheduled surgery, medical or dental procedures should not use the herb for two weeks or more before because it can increase the risk of bleeding. For this reason, blood thinning medications such as aspirin, clopidogrel, ibuprofen, dalteparin, heparin, warfarin, and other similar medications might become more potent than the usual and increase the probability of untoward bleeding.

How to use burdock

Edible burdock roots have been considered a vegetable in the Middle Ages and still continue to be eaten in Japan, Taiwan, and Korea. The roots' crisp, mildly sweet taste and somewhat pungent flavour makes it stand out in soups, stews, and rice dishes. Its undeveloped flower stalks is harvested in late spring and eaten, with a taste reminiscent of artichoke, a related plant. If eaten as food, it can be cooked as a carrot. Beneficial effects can be seen in three weeks but its use has to be limited for two to three months at a time.

Aside from being food, burdock is also available as tincture, teas, or capsules. An ounce of the root and seeds can be decocted to 700 millilitres of water, boiled down to about almost half its volume. It can then be taken in doses of a wineglassful, every six to eight hours daily. Infusion or decoction of the seeds has been given for oedema and other afflictions of the kidney.

Capsules of burdock may be taken at one to two grams every eight hours daily. For those who prefer using the dried root, about two to six grams are steeped in 150 millilitres of boiling water for 15 minutes. After being strained, it can be taken thrice a day or a cloth may be soaked and used as a compress. Tinctures may be given at 1.5 to three drops daily, but it is often combined with other herbs. The same dose may also be given for fluid extracts but taken only twice daily.

Externally, burdock root decoction can be made into a wash for rheumatism, boils, psoriasis, and skin ulcers. Leaves are applied as poultice for tumours and for gout. A tincture and fluid extract of the seeds can also be given for chronic skin conditions.

Studies on burdock

Burdock seeds contain arctigenin and arctiin which has shown potent antiviral properties in mice. It is also an ingredient in essiac for its anti-cancer activity. Arctigenin has anti-inflammatory activities and has memory boosting properties. Arctiin is transformed into oestrogenic metabolites when it passes through the human intestinal bacteria.

Other identified constituents of burdock are inulin, mucilage, sugars, a trace of resin, a mix of fixed and volatile oils, and a dash of tannic acid. It also has a bitter glucoside called lappin. The roots are rich in starch, minerals of calcium and potassium, amino acids, and some derivatives of caffeoylquinic acid. It also has phenolic acids, quercetin and luteolin, that have powerful effect against free radicals.

References:

• Georgetown University Medical Center. "URBAN HERBS: Burdock." 2007. http://pharmacology.georgetown.edu/urbanherbs/burdock.htm (accessed 30 Jun 2013).

• RxList. "Burdock Effectiveness, Safety, and Drug Interactions on RxList." 2013. http://www.rxlist.com/burdock/supplements.htm (accessed 30 Jun 2013).

• The Wild Vegetarian Book. "Burdock." 2011. http://www.wildmanstevebrill.com/Plants.Folder/Burdock.html (accessed 30 Jun 2013).

• Yahoo Health. "What is Burdock? Dosing, Side Effects & More." 2013. http://health.yahoo.net/natstandardcontent/burdock (accessed 30 Jun 2013).

Health from Nature. "Burdock - Arctium lappa | Medicinal use, description and other useful informations about Burdock." 2011. http://health-from-nature.net/Burdock.html (accessed 30 Jun 2013).

CASCARA SAGRADA- Cascara sagrada is a variety of buckthorn whose bark has been used for centuries as a laxative. Its scientific name is Rhamnus purshiana. It is also called cascara buckthorn, bearberry, dogwood, or chittem. The name "cascara sagrada" or sacred bark was given by the Spanish colonizers to honour its potency.

Growing cascara sagrada

This variety of buckthorn is a local plant in North America. It has been found in north California to the Rocky Mountains of Montana to as distant as British Columbia. The cascara sagrada trees are often located by the stream amongst conifer forests. The bark of the cascara is collected early summer or spring, once the bark starts peeling off. Traditionally, it is aged for a year under a shade to retain its typical yellowish hue.

Benefits of cascara sagrada

Cascara sagrada has been used over the years as a laxative for people suffering from constipation. Native Americans have used it for liver problems, expelling gallstones, rheumatism, gonorrhoea, stomach discomfort, and dysentery.

Cascara sagrada bark has been used by the Native Americans of the Pacific Northwest as a purgative. This knowledge was eventually passed on to the Europeans who colonized their territory. In 1999, cascara sagrada had a 20 per cent share in the United States' laxative market with an approximate value of USD 400 million. It's the most extensive herbal ingredient for cathartics today.

Researchers are currently studying cascara sagrada's potential as an antitumor and an antiviral. Its emodin content is said to inhibit the spread of tumor cells although it can be deadly to certain types of cancer cells. In mice, cascara sagrada has shown its ability to inhibit certain viral strains. It has also antibiotic and anti-inflammatory effects. There has yet to be conclusive studies done in humans before it can be used for such indications.

What to look out for

Fresh cascara bark should be treated first otherwise; it will cause violent vomiting and diarrhoea. Using laxatives should not exceed a week or a fortnight (2 Weeks). Long term use might produce dehydration, heart problems, and muscle weakness. They should not be given to children because they have the tendency to lose electrolytes faster.

The use of the cascara sagrada bark has been linked to tummy ache and diarrhoea. In May 2002, the US Food and Drug Administration

(US FDA) banned the use of cascara sagrada in over-the-counter (OTC) laxative medication. By September 20003, cascara has been stricken off the list as an OTC medication. At present, products containing cascara sagrada or any of its components will require a doctor's prescription.

Pregnant and lactating women should also avoid using cascara. It might induce labour or the active components might get passed down to the nursing baby. People with conditions in the intestines, such as Crohn's disease, irritable bowel syndrome, colitis, haemorrhoids, and appendicitis, including those with kidney conditions, should not take cascara sagrada. Expect the urine to taint pink, red, violet, brown, or black.

Some medications might also affect cascara sagrada's effects on the body. Drugs that affect electrolyte balance, such as digoxin, corticosteroids, and diuretics, should be used with caution when taking cascara sagrada. The loss of potassium electrolytes can be devastating on the body. Warfarin and other blood thinners should also be used with caution when taking cascara sagrada. Diarrhoea can increase the risk of bleeding and intensify the potency of these medications, especially warfarin. Do not take cascara sagrada together with another stimulant laxatives, such as bisacodyl, castor oil, senna, and the like.

How to use cascara sagrada

Drink a full glass of water (about 240 millilitres) of water after taking in cascara sagrada or after a meal to lessen the discomfort it might cause. Expect 6 to 12 hours to pass before its effects occur. It is not uncommon that effects might not appear until 24 hours has passed.

Its use as herbal medicine has been associated with cascara sagrada. Other parts may be utilised and consumed as food. The fruits may be eaten but with the usual cathartic effect. Some foods such as soda, liquors, ice cream, and baked products contain food that has cascara as flavouring. It can be applied on the fingernails to stop the habit of nail biting.

The dose for cascara sagrada bark varies from one herbalist to another. It can be as small as 30 grains of powdered bark dissolved in water or about 1 to 3 grams of dried bark. One of the effective doses for the fluid extract is 0.6 to millilitres. In some Scientific studies, a daily amount of 20 to 30 milligrams of the cascaroides are given. For the traditional prescribed amount of cascaroides, one cup of tea is prepared by steeping 2 grams of finely chop up bark placed in 150 millilitres of boiling water for approximately 5 to 10 minutes.

After straining, the liquid extract can be taken for a teaspoonful (about 2 to 5 millilitres) every eight hours. Herbalists will often give the smallest amount of cascara sagrada that will produce soft stools.

Studies on cascara sagrada

The two major active components of cascara sagrada that gave it it's strong cathartic effects are its cascaroides and emodin. Pharmacologically, they are classified as the stimulant type of laxative. Cascaroides trigger peristalsis while emodin provokes the smooth muscle cells of the large intestine.

Chronic use of laxatives has been associated with cancers in the colon and the rectum. However, according to the US FDA, there is no risk for such kind of cancer associated with cascara sagrada. Emodin content from either cascara or aloe has not shown any kind of risk for genetic mutation of live cells either. Any kind of developed mutation might lead to the development of cancer cells.

There is compelling scientific evidence that showed prolonged use of laxatives such as those in cascara sagrada will cause physiological dependence on the bowels. This means the bowels won't be able to move on their own unless a laxative is used to stimulate them. There is also some literature that has linked cascara sagrada use to serious liver conditions.

References:

•   WebMD. "CASCARA." 2009. http://www.webmd.com/vitamins-supplements/ingredientmono-773-

CASCARA.aspx?activeIngredientId=773&activeIngredientName=CA
SCARA (accessed 23 May 2013).

• Drugs.com. "Cascara sagrada." 2013.
http://www.drugs.com/cdi/cascara-sagrada.html (accessed 23 May
2013).

• RxList. "Cascara." 2009.
http://www.rxlist.com/cascara/supplements.htm (accessed 23 May
2013).

• iHerb. "Cascara Sagrada." 2012.
http://healthlibrary.epnet.com/GetContent.aspx?token=e0498803-
7f62-4563-8d47-5fe33da65dd4&chunkiid=625844 (accessed 23
May 2013).

• Sigma Aldritch. "Cascara sagrada."
http://www.sigmaaldrich.com/life-science/nutrition-
research/learning-center/plant-profiler/rhamnus-purshiana.html
(accessed 23 May 2013).

CATNIP- Catnip is an herb that looks like mint but has greyish green leaves. It's known by its scientific name Nepeta cataria or its common names catswort, field balm, or catmint. It's a popular for its effects on cats but it is also beneficial for humans too.

Growing catnip

Catnip is local to Europe and southwest to central Asia. It has small, fragrant flowers that are mostly white with spots of lavender or pink. This plant blooms in late spring up to autumn. Those grown from seeds are rarely nipped by cats compared to those transplanted on plots.

The catnip is often grown as an ornamental plant in gardens. It can attract cats and butterflies and repel aphids and squash bugs. It survives with little water compared to other mints and a lot of sunshine. It can grow to a meter in height and width. Allocate a plot where catnip can be grown at least 20 inches apart and it will not require additional attention.

Benefits of catnip

It acts as an insect and mosquito repellent, better than DEET, an ingredient in most insect repellents. It can be taken as a tea to induce sleep, promote relaxation, and reduce stress. It is also used in cooking. People have used it for migraine, colds, flu, fever, hives, and de-worming although there has yet to be sufficient evidence for it. Smoking catnip is said to elicit a type of marijuana affect. It is used to relieve congestion caused by colds and dry cough.

Whether used as a tea, juice, extract, or dressing, catnip has been employed for a variety of conditions. It may also be given for digestive upset such as indigestion, stomach cramps, bloating, and colic. It used to be a tonic for regulated delayed menstruation and to increase urine flow. Some people believe that applying it directly on the part affected by arthritis or haemorrhoids will relieve the swelling. However, other medications that are more potent have taken instead.

What to look out for

Catnip is relatively safe for a majority of adults. It is unsafe when puffed for recreational use or when taken by mouth in large doses. Children should never be given catnip. Too much ingestion often results in headache and weakness.

Since catnip has been known to stimulate the uterus, it should never be used by pregnant women or those suffering from heavy menstruation. It can also slow down the nervous system so anaesthesia and other anti-anxiety medications given during surgery might be more potent than usual. Avoid catnip a fortnight (Two weeks)before surgery.

Some medications may interact with catnip. People taking lithium should avoid catnip because it allows too much urine to pass and allow lithium to accumulate in the body. Sedatives such as diazepam, phenobarbital, and zolpidem including their derivatives might cause too much sleepiness when used with catnip.

How to use catnip

The leaves and roots of the catnips have opposite actions. Those who drink catnip tea made of flowers will feel relaxed while those made from roots will feel revived. Young leaves are eaten raw in salads. Its leaves and young shoots are used for seasoning in France. Before tea from Asia ever arrived in Europe, the English have been using it as tea. When served cold before meals, it can stimulate the appetite. When taken hot after, it helps aid digestion.

In central Europe, catnip has been used to treat hives, measles and chickenpox. It is believed that catnip will prevent the eruption of blisters and lessen the fever that accompanies it. It has been used as a mild antibiotic and a local anaesthetic. In large doses, it can make anyone vomit.

Traditional doses for catnip involve 2 to 4 grams of dried catnip taken as tea. A 15 per cent nepetalactone essential oil has been found as an insect repellent. According to traditional herbalists, catnip should never be boiled but steeped in boiling water. A teaspoon of catnip to a cup of boiling water should be taken once or twice a day. A more potent preparation is catnip tincture, where half a teaspoon to a full teaspoon is taken. Commercially prepared catnip capsules are taken once or twice daily. Extracts may be taken as tea by mixing 2.5 to 5 millilitres of catnip extract in half a cup of warm water.

When used on skin, the dried catnip flowers or leaves are slightly moistened with warm water. This is then turned into a dressing that is applied as often as needed. Catnip tea when cooled may be used as a soaking bath.

Studies on catnip

The main constituent of catnip is nepetalactone, which is a major component of its essential oil. However, it also contains geranyl, citronellyl, cineol, pinene, and humulene including thymol, camphor, carvacrol, nerol, nepetaside, and other components. It also contains biotin, choline, inositol, manganese, pantothenic acid, including vitamins A and B.

Catnip's effects have been studied in rats. There were reported behavioural changes, decreased functioning, and drowsiness in moderate doses. There are no clinical data to back up catnip's purported effects on the nervous system. There is anecdotal evidence where an infant who consumed large amount of catnip fell into severe depression.

Another study involving guinea pigs and rabbits were able to show catnip's ability to relax the smooth muscles of the trachea and jejunum, similar to that of papaverine. This could explain how catnip tea works but there has yet to be clinical data to support this claim.

Three separate studies using 15 per cent of nepetalactone were able to prove catnip's ability to repel not just mosquitoes but black flies, stable flies, and deer ticks as well. In another separate study, the same concentration of catnip's active ingredient was also able to repel cockroaches.

In 2011, there was a study involving rats and penile erections. According to researchers, rats that consumed food that's made up of 10 per cent catnip leaves were able to improve the rodents' sexual performance by acting on its dopamine dependent systems.

References:

•   The Modern Herbal. "Catnip Herb Health Benefits." 2013. http://themodernherbal.com/2010/12/catnip-herb-health-benefits/ (accessed 27 May 2013).

• Drugs.com. "Catnip." 2009. http://www.drugs.com/npp/catnip.html (accessed 27 May 2013).

• LIVESTRONG. "Benefits of Catnip Tea." 2011. http://www.livestrong.com/article/511243-benefits-of-catnip-tea/ (accessed 27 May 2013).

• Medical health guide. "Catnip Herbal Medicine Uses, Health Benefits, Side Effects." 2011. http://www.medicalhealthguide.com/herb/catnip.htm (accessed 27 May 2013).

• Webmd.com. "CATNIP." 2009. http://www.webmd.com/vitamins-supplements/ingredientmono-831-CATNIP.aspx?activeIngredientId=831&activeIngredientName=CATNIP (accessed 27 May 2013).

CAYENNE- Cayenne pepper is a type of chili pepper with red, slender fruits that are used to add flavour to food. This type of pepper is known as the guinea spice, aleva, or the bird pepper. Its scientific name is Capsicum anuum and is related to paprika and other chilies like the tabasco, bell pepper, and habañero. It's borderline spicy at the Scoville scale.

Growing cayenne

Cayenne peppers grow better in tropical climates with warm, damp, fertile soil. It will take them a quarter of a year to grow.

They can reach heights of 8 inches and taller depending on whether they are bearing peppers (Having pepper on the branch slows the tree's growth) and would need to be spaced twelve inches in between. It grows all year round in South America and in some parts of Asia.

Cayenne peppers have always been a part of tropical cuisine until Christopher Columbus discovered them in the Caribbean. It was introduced around the 15th and 16th century to Europe as a cheaper alternative to the expensive black peppers imported from Asia. Another explorer, Ferdinand Magellan introduced them to

Africa and Asia which used them not just as condiments but also as herbal medicine.

Benefits of cayenne

Despite its spiciness which turns off most people, cayenne is very rich in vitamin A. It also has pyridoxine, riboflavin, vitamins C and E plus minerals like manganese and potassium. A dash of cayenne on food makes these nutritional benefits negligible.

It has been studied for its ability to reduce pain and swelling, it cardiovascular benefits, and its ability to block ulcer formation. It can also relieve nasal congestion. Although its nutrients are barely significant in the diet, cayenne has a very high antioxidant property which makes them effective in controlling damage caused by free radicals. Its heat producing properties may help people lose weight.

What to look out for

Cayenne is a relative of nightshade (Solanaceae) vegetables like eggplant, tomatoes, and potatoes. These plants can aggravate arthritis although there has yet to be a scientific study proving such anecdotal findings.

Use cayenne with caution when taking in anti-asthma medication like theophylline. The herb increases the amount of theophylline absorbed by the body and could lead to overdose or poisoning.

Due to its heat producing ability, people assume that cayenne will further inflame sore tissues. In reality, what it actually does is to imitate the discomfort caused by damage. Garlic, ginger, horseradish, and mustard are herbs that cause actual tissue damage, not cayenne. A topical cream preparation can be used to relieve pain but should not be used on broken skin. There may be initial, nasty sensation during initial application but it eventually disappears over time.

How to use cayenne

The most popular use for cayenne is as spice. Its fruits are dried before being ground and powdered. Most Asian cuisine use cayenne fruits whole in their dishes. A dash of cayenne can be used to any vegetable sauté. Hot cocoa can be made more exciting with a sprinkling of cayenne. Lemon juice mixed with a dash of cayenne complements bitter green vegetables like kale.

Cayenne's active ingredient, capsaicin, reduces pain by depleting substance P. This chemical is produced in the body when there is tissue injury. Initial application will cause a feeling of searing pain but tolerance will eventually develop. A cream made with 0.025% or 0.075% capsaicin content is marketed as a topical analgesic.

Lower concentrations are used to relieve arthritis while higher ones are used for severe cases of neuropathy.

When taken internally, cayenne helps relieve indigestion. It works by depleting substance P to lessen the discomfort. It also protects the stomach from forming ulcers when NSAIDs are used, although its mechanism has yet to be understood. One thing's for sure; it does not kill ulcer-forming bacteria like Heliobacter pylori. A dose of half a teaspoon or 1/4 of a teaspoon thrice a day will relieve dyspepsia.

If used as a gargle for sore throat, 3.5 teaspoon of cayenne powder mixed in 2 cups of boiling water. Cool it down before use.

Local grocers and commercial supermarkets often carry cayenne as a regular mainstay in their shelves. When buying in bulk, keep the cayenne in a tightly sealed glass jar and away from sunlight. Other people prefer to dry them out and pound them to bits before storing them in their kitchen pantries.

Studies on cayenne

The active component of cayenne is found in capsaicin, or 8-methyul-N-vanillyl-6-nonesamide. Scientists have considered its topical use in osteoarthritis, peripheral neuropathy caused by diabetes, post-surgery nerve pain, back pain, psoriasis, and fibromyalgia. It may be taken orally for dyspepsia and to prevent ulcer formation in people who have to take non-steroidal anti-inflammatory drugs (NSAID) for long periods of time. Cayenne may also be given intranasally (In the nose)to relieve rhinitis.

Studies correlating cayenne with dyspepsia were done in 2002 where some participants were given 2,500 milligrams of cayenne per day in divided doses and taken before meals. In the period of five weeks, those who took the said dose found relief from gas, pain, bloating, and nausea.

There is a study conducted in 2009 where patients with rhinitis with unknown cause were made to use nasal sprays that contained 4 micrograms capsaicin thrice daily for a period of three days. These reduced the attacks dramatically. In a 2011 study, a mixture of cayenne and eucalyptus were also used intranasally (In the nose) twice daily for a fortnight (14 days). During that time, the participants were able to obtain relief from sinus congestion and headache.

A 2010 study funded by the National Institutes of Health and the McCormick Spice Company has shown that half a teaspoon, or about 250 milligrams, of cayenne powder mixed in food or taken in its capsulized form was able to burn an additional 10 more calories in four hours in normal weight young adults who have never eaten spicy food before. According to Richard Mattes, professor of foods and nutrition in Purdue University, cayenne seems to irritate the trigeminal nerve on people who are not used to it. Once the body gets used to it, the discomfort wears off.

References:

- Botanical.com. "Cayenne." 1995. http://botanical.com/botanical/mgmh/c/cayenn40.html (accessed 21 May 2013).

- Natural and Alternative Treatments by iHerb. "Cayenne." 2012. healthlibrary.epnet.coma/GetContent.aspx?token=e0498803-7f62-4563-8d47-5fe33da65dd4&chunkiid=21645 (accessed 21 May 2013).

- The World's Healthiest Foods. "Cayenne pepper." 2001. http://www.whfoods.com/genpage.php?tname=foodspice&dbid=140 (accessed 21 May 2013).

- University of Maryland Medical Center . "Cayenne." 2013. http://www.umm.edu/altmed/articles/cayenne--000230.htm (accessed 21 May 2013).

- WebMD. "Cayenne Pepper May Burn Calories, Curb Appetite." 2010. http://www.webmd.com/diet/news/20110427/cayenne-pepper-may-burn-calories-curb-appetite (accessed 21 May 2013).

CHAMOMILE- Chamomile is an herb that has been used as tea to promote calm sleep. The name comes from the Greek word "chamaimelon' which means earth apple. The British spell it as camomile. It became more popular in the Middle Ages where it was the European ginseng. Up to this day, chamomile is included as a drug in 26 pharmacopoeias. Chamomile is also known as bodegold, manzanilla, pin heads, and maythen.

Growing chamomile

There are two types of chamomile being used in herbal treatments. Matricaria chamomile or the German chamomile, and the Chamaemelum nobile or the English chamomile. Although two different species, these share the same components which made them valuable herbal medication.

Various species of chamomile can be found all throughout Europe, North Africa, and some temperate areas of Asia. Some species grows best on dry, sandy soil in a sunny environment while others prefer moist, black, loam. Seeds are often sown in May and eventually transplanted, though it's not recommended as double flowered varieties work better as herbal medication. Because of this, old plants are divided by sets in March with rows 2.5 feet apart and 1.5 feet in between. Others prefer to divide the sets in autumn because it will thrive better.

Benefits of chamomile

Chamomile has been used clinically to treat stress and insomnia. Other potential benefits are its antiseptic and anti-microbial properties. It also prevents inflammation and can prevent ulcer formation by altering the amount of pepsin being secreted. It also has some blood thinning properties and can regulate high blood glucose. When used as a cosmetic, chamomile extracts can retain moisture and prevent swelling.

The wild or German chamomile has been known to treat women's condition such as premenstrual syndrome (PMS) or menstrual cramps. It can relieve spasms of smooth muscles which can relieve gas and bloating, especially in colicky babies or irritable children. It can also keep tics and twitching at a minimum. Although it promotes sleep, it will not interfere with tasks that require concentration and focus, compared to chemical sedatives.

What to look out for

Very few people have developed an allergy for chamomile, except for those allergic to ragweed and other related plants such as chrysanthemums, daisies, or marigold. Those who do might experience skin rashes, breathlessness, and a swollen throat. Chamomile use might actually make asthma worse. It also has oestrogen-like effects so women with hormone-sensitive cancers should never take it.

There are risks when using chamomile. It contains some coumarin, a natural blood thinner. Stop chamomile use when scheduled for surgery in a fortnight (Two weeks) to prevent undue bleeding. The herb can also interact with other medications such as sedatives, blood thinners, and non-steroidal anti-inflammatory drugs (NSAID). Herbs such as ginkgo biloba, garlic, saw palmetto, St. John's wort, and valerian may potentiate chamomile's blood thinning and sedating effects.

Chamomile might also lower blood pressure and blood sugar. Anti-diabetic and medications for hypertension might be further potentiated. Since chamomile is also broken down by some enzymes in the liver so drugs such as fexofenadine, oral contraceptives, and some antifungals might also be affected.

Most experts believe that chamomile is safe for pregnant and nursing women. However, long term use of chamomile has not been studied extensively.

How to use chamomile

Chamomile has a brilliant blue volatile oil known as chamazulene. This very potent oil is a very potent anti-inflammatory which can be placed on skin infections. Another alternative would be to soak a cloth in strong chamomile tea and use as patch on eczema and other similar skin conditions. It also has anthemic acid, which gives it a slightly bitter aftertaste.

For children affected with skin rashes or itchy insect bites, four tablespoons of chamomile flowers with half a cup of oatmeal in an old stocking should do the trick. Secure it with elastic under the bathtub's spigot before filling the tub. Have them bathe as usual. Suggested doses for children are usually half of the adult dose but those younger than five should never take more than a cup. To relieve colic, 30 to 60 millilitre of the tea may be given per day.

There is no standard dose for chamomile. Research on the herb's effects used 400 to 1,600 milligrams per day in a capsule. The most common use for chamomile is to take as a tea. Infuse a tablespoon of chamomile flowers for every cup of water for 15 minutes. Drink 120 millilitres every four to five hours for digestive complaints or mix with equal parts of hops or skullcap for nervous problems. The tea may be used as a gargle or mouthwash for sore throat and swollen gums.

Tincture of chamomile contains one part of the essential oil dissolved in five parts of alcohol. About 30 to 60 drops of the tincture may be dissolved in hot water and taken every eight hours. The essential oil may be inhaled by putting a few drops of it in hot water. Breathe in the steam to relieve cough. Used chamomile tea bags or cloth soaked in chamomile tea may be used to soothe sore, painful eyes.

Studies on chamomile

Chamomile has chemicals that have the ability to bind to the gamma amino butyric acid (GABA) receptors which helps control monoamine neurotransmitters. When regulated, it will promote relaxation and a feeling of peacefulness. Researchers have yet to determine which specific chemical does this.

However, there very clinical studies done on people to have any documented evidence it is good for any specific condition. There are some earlier studies that showed it possible potential to provide relief from mouth ulcers caused by chemotherapy or radiation.

There is insufficient evidence that can show chamomile as an effective herbal medication for travel sickness, attention deficit hyperactivity disorder (ADHD), fibromyalgia, and hay fever.

There is a German study that showed chamomile's microbial properties. Its constituents were able to inactivate toxins produced by the bacteria, specifically Staphylococci and Streptococci strains. Its effects become more potent when combined with other herbal antimicrobials such as thyme, echinacea, and goldenseal.

References:

- Herb Wisdom. "Chamomile Benefits & Information." 2013. http://www.herbwisdom.com/herb-chamomile.html (accessed 3 Jun 2013).

- N.D., Jennifer. "Discovery Health "Chamomile: Herbal Remedies"." 2013. http://health.howstuffworks.com/wellness/natural-medicine/herbal-remedies/chamomile-herbal-remedies.htm (accessed 3 Jun 2013).

- National Center for Complementary and Alternative Medicine (NCCAM). "Chamomile | NCCAM." 2007. http://nccam.nih.gov/health/chamomile/ataglance.htm (accessed 3 Jun 2013).

- University of Maryland Medical Center. "German chamomile." 2012. http://www.umm.edu/altmed/articles/german-chamomile-000232.htm (accessed 3 Jun 2013).

- WebMD. "Chamomile: Herbal Information From WebMD." 2012. http://www.webmd.com/vitamins-and-supplements/lifestyle-guide-11/supplement-guide-chamomile (accessed 3 Jun 2013).

CINNAMON- Cinnamon is a herbal seasoning from the Cinnamomum trees that is used to spice up sweet and flavoursome dishes. There are many types of cinnamon being sold on the market today. There's the Cinnamomum verum or the true cinnamon, and the rest are referred to as cassia. The name cinnamon comes from the Greek word "kinamōmon." In some European languages the word comes from the Latin word "canella," a shortened term for tube, as cinnamon bark has the tendency to curl up when it dries up.

Growing cinnamon

Cinnamon has been used in antiquity. It was introduced to Egyptians around 2000 BC. It had been mentioned in the Bible and the Torah as one of the important spices that was used as incense and perfume. It was often given as gifts to kings and offerings to the gods. During that time, cinnamon was cultivated mainly in Bangladesh, Sri Lanka, and Burma. By 1796, the demand for Ceylon's cinnamon had waned as the cheaper cassia became more tolerable to consumers. At present, Sri Lanka produces 80 per cent of the world's supply of cinnamon, with the remaining in Madagascar and Seychelles. Other species of cinnamon, the cassia variety, is grown mostly in Indonesia. About one third of the world's cassia supply comes from China, India, and Vietnam.

The tree can grow to about 30 feet and will have leathery leaves and small yellow flowers. To get the most out of the cinnamon bark, the two year old cinnamon tree is cut near the ground until shoots come out from its roots. Its branches will have its outer bark scraped off to get to the inner bark. True cinnamon will have a light tan color, a very fragrant scent, and subtle flavour.

Benefits of cinnamon

Cinnamon bark is used in folk medicine to clean wounds, release stomach gas, and as an astringent. It's a traditional home remedy for diarrhoea, nausea, indigestion, and poor appetite. Its warmth has been used as a basis for treating colds and cold extremities. Newer studies have shown cinnamon to have anti-diabetic and anti-microbial aside from its antioxidant effect. Its effects on blood glucose have also been attributed to its weight loss effect.

What to look out for

There is occasional incidence of allergic reactions for cinnamon bark tea. The allergy will appear as increased sweating accompanied by quick, shallow breathing and drowsiness following extreme agitation. Cinnamon oil is often highly concentrated and is very poisonous. It will cause stomach upset and kidney damage when taken internally. When rubbed on skin, the oil will cause burning and redness.

About 0.45 per cent of coumarin is found in the cassia variety and little or none in true cinnamon. That makes them possibly unsafe when taken for long periods of time. It might worsen or even cause liver disease. Avoid using it with other herbal medications that could affect the liver such as kava, pennyroyal, comfrey, and germander. Be careful also when using cinnamon with other herbs that can lower blood sugar such as bitter gourd, fenugreek, garlic, ginseng, and psyllium.

An experiment showed that cinnamon extract can affect the absorption of tetracycline. Clinical studies have yet to be done to prove its effects on humans. Another experimental data bared that cinnamon extract can cause malformation in the young of rats and chick embryos.

How to use cinnamon

Adding cinnamon to food is one of the most common uses of this plant. It's mixed in with tea, cocoa, and liqueurs or in meat dishes. Cassia is often used in sweets. Some cultures use cinnamon sticks for pickling. Mediterranean cuisine puts cinnamon in their soups, desserts, and drinks.

Ancient doctors used cinnamon to treat snake bites, colds, and some kidney conditions. Egyptians have used it to embalm their mummies. Extracts from the leaves can be used as mosquito repellent, although some use the extract to kill mosquito larvae in stagnant water.

When using cinnamon as a digestive, a teaspoon of ground bark can be steeped in hot water and taken as tea. Alternatively, 15 to 30 drops of liquid cinnamon extract may be dissolved in a glass of water. Cinnamon powder may be mixed with honey and used as a spread on bread to benefit from its insulin regulating effects. Cinnamon oil is used for aromatherapy and should not be taken internally or applied on the skin.

Average dose of the herbal medication is at 2000 to 4000 milligrams in divided doses. Any form of cinnamon should be placed in a tight glass or metal container that will protect it from exposure to light and excessive moisture.

Studies on cinnamon

Cinnamon's flavour and aroma is caused by an essential oil that makes up 0.5 to 1 per cent of the bark's components. The golden yellow essential oil is made up of cinnamic aldehyde that forms 90 per cent of the extract. It may also contain traces of coumarin, ethyl cinnamate, eugenol, beta-caryophylline, linalool, and methyl chavicol. In the leaves, compounds such as cinnamyl acetate, eugenol, anethole, and some traces of cinnamaldehyde were found.

A study conducted in 2000 showed that the extract of Cinnamomum cassia had a significant effect on Human Immunodeficiency Virus type I. In another experiment in 2008, Cinnamomum vera showed substantial antiviral effects, although it was done with silkworm cells. Aside from viruses, a substance in cinnamon is detected by Japanese researchers that could prevent certain strains of fungi, Staphylococci, Clostridium, and Escherichia.

Two studies in 2008 and 2012 have confirmed extracts of cinnamon included in the diet will help improve blood glucose levels in type II diabetics.

Like other herbal medications, cinnamon has also been studied for cancer. According to a 2010 study, cinnamaldehyde was able to trigger an antioxidant effect in the lining of the colon which makes them effective in preventing colon cancer. In an earlier study, cinnamaldehyde was found to prevent skin cancer.

A significant breakthrough research in 2011 involved a cinnamon extract which was able to inhibit the development of Alzheimer's disease in rats.

References:

• Encyclopedia of Life. "Cinnamomum verum: Cinnamon." 2012. http://eol.org/pages/490672/overview (accessed 21 May 2013).

- Health from Nature. "CINNAMON - Cinnamomum zeylanicum." 2011. http://health-from-nature.net/Cinnamon.html (accessed 21 May 2013).

- Herbal Information. "Cinnamomum verum J.S. Presl. (Lauraceae)." 2008. http://herbalinformation.awardspace.com/?cm=c&fn=cinnamomum_verum (accessed 21 May 2013).

- Herbal Remedies. "Cinnamon." 2000. http://www.herbalremedies.com/cinnamon-information.html (accessed 21 May 2013).

- Medline Plus. "Cassia cinnamon." 2012. http://www.nlm.nih.gov/medlineplus/druginfo/natural/1002.html (accessed 21 May 2013).

CRANBERRY- Cranberry is an evergreen creeping shrub whose deep red berries are used as one of the common herbal medication for kidney and bladder conditions. It is often found as juice, sauce, jam, or sweetened dried berries. They are called bearberry, mossberry, fenberry, atoca, bounceberry or sassamanash. The name comes from its flowers which resembled a crane's head and neck. Vaccinium oxycoccos, Vaccinium erythrocarpum, and Vaccinium macrocarpon are some of the species of cranberry utilised for its health benefits

Growing cranberry

Cranberries are a major commercial crop in Wisconsin, United States and British Columbia, Canada. The shrubs grow from one to four inches high with extensive vines. The leaves appear green and maroon when young but turn olive green when mature. Light pink flowers appear in clusters by mid-summer before turning into berries. Although the plant prefers full sun or light shade, it's sturdy enough to withstand extreme drops in temperature.

Since cranberries grow on wetlands, commercial producers utilise cranberry beds which are often flooded to simulate similar conditions. These berries are propagated by transferring vines from an old bed to another. By June to July, pink flowers that bloom become berries. From September to November, cranberries are harvested. Wet harvesting is done for most preparation of cranberries while dry handpicked cranberries are done for those sold as whole berries in the market.

Benefits of cranberry

Cranberry has been used by the Native American Indians for urinary conditions. In fact, the extracted juice can actually prevent, but not treat, infections in the urinary tract. It has also been used for controlling type II diabetes, chronic fatigue syndrome (CFS), scurvy, pleurisy, ulcers, and some cancers. It's rich in salicylic acid which lessens swelling, promotes blood thinning, and has possible anti-tumour properties.

What to look out for

The Committee on Safety of Medicines in the United Kingdom issued a warning in 2004 that advised patients not to take cranberry when they're on warfarin. This was due to the increased incidence of bruising caused by the presence of salicylic acid in cranberries. However, a 2006 review revealed that the bruising is associated in people in a certain gene.

For most people, cranberry juice and extracts are safe, even for children. Consuming the fresh berries and the juice are also safe for breastfeeding and pregnant women. Dietary supplements that contain cranberry have yet to prove their safety for women with these conditions.

Drinking too much of the juice can cause slight stomach discomfort and diarrhoea. More than a litre's worth of cranberry juice per day can cause stone formation in the kidneys. The juice contains high amounts of oxalate which can combine with calcium to form kidney stones.

There are some medications that could interact with cranberry. Cranberry can affect the time how the liver breaks down medications. This increases the risk for potentially harmful side effects. Such medications to look out for are diazepam, and other similar medications.

How to use cranberry

Cranberry juice is the most consumed preparation from cranberries. However, since the berries are naturally sour with a bitter aftertaste, most manufacturers often add a teaspoon of sweetener per ounce. That makes the cranberry juice more sugar laden than the regular soda. To get the most out of cranberries, fresh berries bought from the store can be frozen where it will keep for up to nine months. About 1.5 kilos of fresh cranberries can yield about a litre of 100 per cent pure cranberry juice. The ones bought at the grocer's is made up of 26 to 33 per cent of cranberry juice only.

To prevent UTIs in adults, one to 10 ounces of cranberry juice per day has been used. About 1.5 ounces of fresh or frozen fruit may also be given for this condition. For children, a tablespoon for every kilo of their weight may be given. To deodorize the urine in incontinent patients, three to six ounces per day may be given. For those with type II diabetes, six capsules or about 240 millilitres of the juice may be given per day for three months. For people who want to increase the amount of good bacteria in their digestive tract, two ounces of cranberry juice for three months will suffice.

There are data which supports the use of cranberry juice and supplements in preventing urinary tract infections. However, there is very little evidence that shows it's effective for controlling type II diabetes' blood sugar. More data is needed to prove cranberry's success in treating benign prostatic hyperplasia (BPH), speed up skin healing, pleurisy, cancers, and CFS.

Studies on cranberry

There was a 2005 research that showed cranberry juice contains dense molecules of non-diffusible substance which could prevent formation of plaque in teeth. This is done by inhibiting Streptococcus mutans, major bacteria that can cause tooth decay. This ability of cranberry juice to prevent adhesion on living tissues has made it a valuable aid in preventing infections in the bladder and the urethra.

A 2010 study showed that the tannins present in cranberries have blood thinning properties and could prevent urinary tract infections (UTI) from recurring in women. Two years after, data review and more trials were able to show that it cannot prevent UTIs from frequently occurring as there is long term tolerance. In fact, data from 2002 and 2003 studies showed that cranberry juice might contribute to calcium oxalate stone formation in the kidneys. A latest 2013 study revealed that these tannins in cranberry can interact with proteins and digestive enzymes that could affect how starch is hydrolysed. This is a potential weight loss benefit that has yet to be verified in trials.

In a 2011 study, cranberry juice was able to reduce bad cholesterol and increase antioxidant activity in the blood in eight weeks compared to placebo. However, this wasn't enough to improve hypertension, cholesterol, and blood sugar levels in the blood. There is are preliminary research data in 2013 that showed cranberry juice consumption in type II diabetic patients might actually lower their blood sugar levels.

References:

• Herbal Supplement Resource. "Cranberry - Side Effects and Benefits." 2006. http://www.herbal-supplement-resource.com/cranberry-herb.html (accessed 4 Jun 2013).

• Medical health guide. "Cranberry, Herbal Medicine - Uses, Health Benefits, Side Effects." 2002.

http://www.medicalhealthguide.com/herb/cranberry.htm (accessed 4 Jun 2013).

- National Centre for Complementary and Alternative Medicine (NCCAM). "Cranberry | NCCAM." 2005. http://nccam.nih.gov/health/cranberry (accessed 4 Jun 2013).

- University of Maryland Medical Centre. "Cranberry." 2012. http://www.umm.edu/altmed/articles/cranberry-000235.htm (accessed 4 Jun 2013).

- WebMD. "CRANBERRY: Uses, Side Effects, Interactions and Warnings - WebMD." 2009. http://www.webmd.com/vitamins-supplements/ingredientmono-958-CRANBERRY.aspx?activeIngredientId=958&activeIngredientName=CRANBERRY (accessed 4 Jun 2013).

DANDELION- The dandelion is a flowering herb that is found in temperate regions and is often considered as a weed growing in lawns, on roadsides, and shores. They are known for their yellow flowery heads that turns into silver tufts that blow into the wind. Its scientific name is Taraxacum officinale and is also known as lion's tooth, cankerwort, milk witch, Irish daisy, and wild endive.

Growing dandelion

Dandelions come from a single taproot and extend into numerous stems that can grow from 16 to 28 inches tall. Its roots are dark brown, somewhat fleshy, and filled with bitter, smelly, milk-like latex. The slender stems are somewhat purple and have flower heads at the end. The fruits are the ends of the silver tufts. Each flowering head can produce about 54 to 172 seeds which are propagated wherever the wind blows. The flowers open in full sunlight and close at night or gloomy weather. It's a native plant in Eurasian regions but have been naturalized in the Americas, South Africa, Australia, and New Zealand. The whole plant is used and is often harvested early in spring.

Benefits of dandelion

Although many gardeners consider the dandelion a pesky weed, it actually has culinary and medicinal benefits. Native Americans have long utilized the plant both as food and medicine. Its flowers are used for wine-making; the greens are made into salads and soups, while the roots act as non-caffeinated substitute for coffee.

As an herbal medication, dandelions have been used as a mild laxative, improve appetite, and enhance digestion. Its milk-like latex has been employed as mosquito repellent and home remedy for warts. In Chinese medicine, dandelion has been used to treat problems of the digestive tract and to improve milk flow or relieve soreness. In Europe, dandelions are the herbal remedy for fever, boils, diabetes, diarrhea, and eye conditions. Arabic medicine has used it as a tonic for major internal organs.

Other benefits that can be derived from dandelion is its ability to relieve joint and muscle pains, eczema, and bruises. Its toning effects are believed to benefit the skin, blood, and digestive tract. Some people swear by its ability to treat viral infections and some cancers.

At present, the dandelion has been used for liver and gallbladder conditions as well as appetite stimulant. The leaves are used as a diuretic, especially for those affected with edema. Herbalists claim that it also improves kidney function.

What to look out for

Dandelions are generally considered safe, especially when taken as food. However, some people have developed allergies to it and might develop mouth sores upon its ingestion. People allergic to chrysanthemums, marigold, chamomile, yarrow, daisies, and iodine should stay clear of dandelions. Some people may develop heartburn and hyperacidity when consuming dandelion. It may also irritate their skin.

Since dandelion is a diuretic, it can affect how fast any drug can leave the body. This might render some medications, such as antacids and ciprofloxacin, useless. Other drugs, such as blood thinners, diuretics, lithium, and anti-diabetics, might actually become more potent and become more harmful than usual.

Drugs that are affected by liver metabolism may also be affected by dandelion consumption because it might slow down or hasten how the liver usually breaks down the medication. Drugs such as haloperidol, odansetron, propranolol, theophylline and the like might have increased incidence of harmful side effects. On the other hand, acetaminophen, atorvastatin, diazepam, digoxin, lamotrigine, morphine, and other similar drugs might be rendered inactive.

How to use dandelion

Leaves of the dandelions can be eaten raw in salads or cooked as soups. Young leaves and buds that have yet to bloom are eaten as salads while the older leaves are cooked. It tastes similar to mustard greens, so raw leaves have a somewhat bitter taste. Salads made from dandelion leaves come with hard boiled eggs. The flowers have been used in wines, ale, and soda. Another preparation with flowers involves using them as a jam. Dandelion flower heads are mixed with lemon to make a honey substitute that has medicinal value. Harvest those dandelions growing in good, fertile soil and make sure to wash them thoroughly and steer clear from those that might have contact with dangerous pesticides.

Dandelion roots are recognised as a drug in Canada where it is used as a diuretic. The supplements are sold fresh or dried. It can also be sold as tinctures, liquid extracts, teas, capsules, and tablets. Ask a health professional if children are to use such supplement. Since there are no standard doses for dandelion as herbal medicine, traditional doses have to be tweaked by a health professional to respond to your condition.

Dried dandelion leaves are steeped for five to 10 minutes in hot water and taken thrice a day at a teaspoonful or two. Chopped, dried dandelion roots are cooked in boiling water for five to 10 minutes and drained before being taken at 2.5 to 10 millilitres every eight hours. Leaf and root tinctures are taken at 30 to 60 drops dissolved in a glass of water and drank once to thrice a day. Powdered extracts are often 500 milligrams

Studies on dandelion

The leaves of the dandelion are rich in vitamins A, B complex, C, and D as well as minerals such as iron, potassium, and zinc. It also contains inulin and levulin, complex starches that help balance blood sugar. It also has taraxacin, a bitter substance that can promote digestion and stimulate the flow of bile from the liver. There is choline in its roots which act as liver tonic and great for detoxification. Scientists believe that the dandelion works by having chemicals that can prevent inflammation and increase urine flow. Its exact mechanism is still unknown.

Although the dandelion has been used for a variety of conditions, there are insufficient evidence that can show its effectiveness in preventing urinary tract infections (UTI), improving appetite, relieving gastro-intestinal conditions such as stomach upset, gas, bloating, or constipation, and in relieving pain similar to arthritis.

References:

• Discovery Health. ""Dandelion: Herbal Remedies"." 2007. http://health.howstuffworks.com/wellness/natural-medicine/herbal-remedies/dandelion-herbal-remedies.htm (accessed 5 Jun 2013).

• Medline Plus. "Dandelion: MedlinePlus Supplements." 2006. http://www.nlm.nih.gov/medlineplus/druginfo/natural/706.html (accessed 5 Jun 2013).

• National Center for Complementary and Alternative Medicine (NCCAM). "Dandelion | NCCAM." 2006. http://nccam.nih.gov/health/dandelion (accessed 5 Jun 2013).

- University of Maryland Medical Center. "Dandelion." 2012. http://www.umm.edu/altmed/articles/dandelion-000236.htm (accessed 5 Jun 2013).

- WebMD. "DANDELION: Uses, Side Effects, Interactions and Warnings - WebMD." 2012. http://www.webmd.com/vitamins-supplements/ingredientmono-706-DANDELION.aspx?activeIngredientId=706&activeIngredientName=DANDELION (accessed 5 Jun 2013).

ECHINACEA- Echinacea is a genus of coneflowers that have been utilised for its ability to boost the body's resistance to disease. There are three species known for their medicinal properties: Echinacea angustifolia, Echinacea pallida, and Echinacea purpurea. Those sold in the market may contain different species or a mix of these. The term Echinacea comes from the Greek word "echino," meaning sea urchin because of its flowers' spiny central disc. It's also known by its common names black Susan, comb flower, coneflower, Indian head, Kansas Snakeroot, and red sunflower.

Growing Echinacea

Echinacea is an herb native to North America where they are often found in prairies and open woodlands. They are grown from seeds and will germinate in a week or two. It has large colorful flowers that bloom from early to late summer. These plants can tolerate drought but different species react differently to elevation and temperature changes.

Benefits of Echinacea

Many herbalists believe that Echinacea can stimulate the body's immune system and ward off infections. In fact, American Indians of the plains used this for its medicinal properties. It has been used for coughs, sore throats, headaches, and management of pain.

Aside from colds, Echinacea in addition is also used for urinary tract infections (UTI), flu, as well as yeast infections of the vagina, bacterial infections of the reproductive tract, diphtheria, malaria, and typhoid. Some people even use Echinacea for chronic fatigue syndrome (CFS), joint pain, migraine, vertigo, and ADHD (Attention Deficit-Hyperactivity Disorder). Other conditions that have benefited from Echinacea are skin conditions such as boils, eczema, burns, ulcers, wounds, sunburn, psoriasis, as well as bee stings, herpes simplex, and Hemorrhoids.

What to look out for

When used short term, Echinacea is likely safe although there is very little information about its long term use. However, since this herb affects the immune system, people with auto-immune conditions such as multiple sclerosis, systemic lupus Erythematosus (SLE), rheumatoid arthritis (RA) and other similar conditions should steer clear of it.

Echinacea is generally safe. However, there are some reported side effects which are rare and reversible. Most of the side effects appear in the skin and in the gastrointestinal tract. Nausea, abdominal pain, diarrhea, itching, and rashes are some of the most common side effects that are associated with using Echinacea. Other side effects associated with the use of Echinacea are bitter aftertaste, numbness of the tongue, dry mouth, insomnia, and muscle aches.

Other medications might also interact with Echinacea. It could slow down how the body breaks down caffeine. It can also affect drugs that require liver metabolism in order to be active in the body. Patients taking medications such as lovastatin, clarithromycin, cyclosporine, diltiazem, indinavir, haloperidol, imipramine, olanzapine, zileuton, propranol and the like should let their physicians know if they intend to use Echinacea. The effects of immunosuppressants such as azathioprine, tacrolumus, corticosteroids and other similar drugs might be lessened when taken with echinacea.

Since supplements are not scrutinised by the US Food and Drugs Administration (US FDA), Echinacea supplements available in the market may have questionable quality. These products are often mislabeled, even those that claim to be standardized, these might not contain any Echinacea at all. Others may be contaminated with poisonous levels of lead and arsenic.

Echinacea how to use it

Two of the most common uses of Echinacea are for the common cold and to relieve vaginal yeast infections. Taking Echinacea at the first sign of a cold you might be able to moderately reduce its symptoms and even shorten its duration. There has yet to be compelling evidence to show Echinacea can actually prevent colds in adults. When stricken with yeast infections, using topical Econazole cream and taking Echinacea is believed to reduce the probability of having it again by 16 per cent.

Some people have used Echinacea for herpes of the genital area. A dose of 800 milligrams of Echinacea extract taken twice a day for half a year was not able to prevent, reduce its recurrence, or even shorten its duration. Additional evidence may needed for Echinacea's use against UTIs, migraine, CFS, eczema, bee stings, ADHD, and flu.

The roots, flowers, and leaves are the plant parts used in Echinacea. Commercial products may come as tablets, juice or tea. There are varied doses in different preparations that contain Echinacea. Freeze dried Echinacea juice extracts contain 100 milligrams and taken every eight hours. The juice of purpurea species may be given at a daily dose of six to nine millilitres for up to eight weeks. These varied formulations of Echinacea should never be used at the same time to prevent overdose.

Studies on Echinacea

Some of the identified Echinacea active components are its chicoric acid, caftaric acid, and echinacoside. It has been listed in the United States National Formulary from 1916 to 1950 but has been removed due to lack of evidence and popularity of antibiotics was at its peak.

The Maryland University did a earlier review on Echinacea in 1997 and it was based on thirteen European research studies that revealed that when Echinacea was taken by people with colds, the symptoms were reduced as well as its duration. Because of the reviews, Europe's Medicines Agency (EMA) approved the expressed juice that come from the flowering heads of the E. purpurea's use as short term treatment and prevention of the ordinary colds.

A 2003 study done by the University of Virginia stated that Echinacea extracts have no significant medicinal value. Two years after, a manufacturer of Echinacea supplements called that study erroneous because instead of 3000 milligrams per day, the study used less than a gram in its trials. There is a 2007 study that state that Echinacea can cut the chances of catching a cold in half and shorten its duration to a day and a half. Experts disagree because the research lacked definitive results. According to the literature reviews done in 2006 to 2009, researchers have been able to conclude that there is a great lack of controlled trials that studied Echinacea's effects on the immune system.

References:

• 	Drugs.com. "Echinacea medical facts from Drugs.com." 1996. http://www.drugs.com/mtm/echinacea.html (accessed 5 Jun 2013).

• 	Mayo Clinic. "Echinacea (Echinacea angustifolia, Echinacea pallida, Echinacea purpurea) - MayoClinic.com." 2012.

http://www.mayoclinic.com/health/echinacea/NS_patient-echinacea (accessed 5 Jun 2013).

- RxList. "Echinacea Effectiveness, Safety, and Drug Interactions on RxList." 2013. http://www.rxlist.com/echinacea/supplements.htm (accessed 5 Jun 2013).

- WebMD. "ECHINACEA: Uses, Side Effects, Interactions and Warnings - WebMD." 2009. http://www.webmd.com/vitamins-supplements/ingredientmono-981-ECHINACEA.aspx?activeIngredientId=981&activeIngredientName=ECHINACEA (accessed 5 Jun 2013).

- University of Maryland Medical Center. "Echinacea." 2012. http://www.umm.edu/altmed/articles/echinacea-000239.htm (accessed 5 Jun 2013).

EUCALYPTUS- Eucalyptus is the genus of tall trees that are rich in volatile oil known as eucalyptol. The world's source of eucalyptus oil comes from the Eucalyptus globulus also known as the blue gum, fever tree, gully gum, or the Tasmanian blue gum. Its name came from the blue wax that covers its leaves.

Growing eucalyptus

The eucalyptus tree is one of the most popular trees cultivated in Australia. They are known as main fodder for koalas. These can grow from 30 to 55 metres tall which are natives of Tasmania and southern parts of Victoria in Australia. Some areas in southern Europe, South Africa, New Zealand, and even to the western regions of the United States to the islands of Hawaii have eucalyptus trees that have been harvested for their eucalyptol, terpenes, and aroma.

The eucalyptus tree is known for its bark that strips often. The narrow, shiny, sickle shaped, dark green leaves are found alternately on rounded stems and opposite each other in squarish ones. Its flowers are cream colored and produce nectar that can be used as honey. The fruits are somewhat woody and have many seeds. The roots grow deep.

Benefits of eucalyptus

The oil from eucalyptus has been used by Australian aborigines to treat wounds and to cure fungal infections. The leaves are made into teas that are said to reduce fevers. Eventually, traditional Chinese, Ayurvedic, and Greek medicine incorporated this plant as one of their herbal medications.

Eucalyptus leaves have been used for a variety of infections, stomach upset, and to get rid of stubborn phlegm in dry cough. Its effects in the upper respiratory system have made it valuable for conditions such as whooping cough, asthma, and tuberculosis in the lungs. It has also been used for joint problems such as osteoarthritis and rheumatism. Some people have used it on the skin for burns, slow healing ulcers, acne, ringworm, and wounds. It has been employed to relieve liver and gallbladder problems, stimulate the appetite, and cancer. The constituents of its leaves may have anti-diabetic properties which keep blood glucose spikes in check.

What to look out for

The oils of the eucalyptus should never be taken or used without being diluted. Pure eucalyptus oil is dangerous, as 3.5 millilitres can kill. Poisoning due to eucalyptus oil may appear as pain in the stomach, dizziness, muscle weakness, narrow eye pupils, and difficulty breathing.

Eucalyptus leaves are generally safe when taken in small amounts in food. As a chemical, eucalyptol can be used as medicine (when diluted) and ingested for as long as three months. For children, eucalyptus is unsafe. Anything larger than what can be taken as food should never be given to children.

Eucalyptol has the ability to affect blood glucose levels. People who are taking maintenance medications for diabetes should monitor their blood glucose levels regularly lest it dips too low. Same goes for people who have to undergo surgery in a fortnight. Stop using anything with eucalyptus a week or two before surgery.

Medicines that pass through the liver are also affected by eucalyptus. The plant extracts might slow down how the liver breaks down the medications. Drugs such as haloperidol, odansetron, verapamil, lansoprazole, nelfinavir, ibuprofen, warfarin, glipizide, losartan and other similar drugs might have an increased risk for side effects. Talk to a health professional first before ever using eucalyptus in any treatment regimen.

Herbs rich in pyrrolizidine alkaloids might damage the liver. Using eucalyptus with herbs such as borage, butterbur, coltsfoot, forget-me-not, ragwort and the like might make it more toxic.

How to use eucalyptus

Diluted eucalyptus oil may be applied on the skin as an insect repellent and to relieve specific joints that are swollen and painful. Another alternative way of using eucalyptus oil is to apply it near the throat or the nostrils to allow the volatile oils to be inhaled. Eucalyptus oil may also be mixed with equal parts of apple cider vinegar and used as antiseptic on wounds, boils, and insect bites.

About five drops of the oil are recognised as a therapeutic dose in the United States Pharmacopoeia. An ointment using eucalyptus oil as its ingredient is listed in the British Pharmacopoeia. For topical use, an ounce of the oil is mixed with a pint of lukewarm water and applied on ulcers and sores. A dose of half a teaspoon to a teaspoonful of the fluid extract have been used for scarlet fever, typhoid, and sporadic fever.

Eucalyptus has been an ingredient in lozenges, syrups, rubs, and even vapours baths to relieve cough and colds. Fresh leaves in teas and gargles have been prescribed by herbalists to alleviate sore throat and heal upper respiratory conditions such as sinusitis and bronchitis. The cineole-rich eucalyptus oil is an antiseptic that can kill bacteria that cause bad breath, plaque, and gingivitis.

There are insufficient scientific studies on the claims that eucalyptus oil can actually reduce the inflammation of the windpipe, relieve stuffy nose, heal wounds, burns, or ulcers fast, control blood glucose spikes in diabetics, improve appetite, and relieve joint pain.

Adults using eucalyptus oil may dissolve 15 to 30 drops to half a cup of sesame, almond, or olive oil before it can be applied on the skin. If the oil is for inhalation, put five to 10 drops of eucalyptus oil in two cups boiling water before placing the towel over your head and inhale the skin.

Studies on eucalyptus

Cineol (also known as eucalyptol), pinene, limonene, citronellal, cryptine, and piperitone are some of the major components that are derived in eucalyptus extracts, aside from the other compounds. The smell of the essential oil is somewhat similar to camphor, only more pungent and sharp.

According to research, eucalyptol from eucalyptus oil has the ability to break up components of viscous phlegm. Asthmatics that have used eucalyptol have been able to lower their corticosteroids. However, since there is not enough study on how eucalyptol does this, patients must ask their healthcare provider's opinion on its use.

References:

• Discovery Health. ""Aromatherapy: Eucalyptus"." 2007. http://health.howstuffworks.com/wellness/natural-medicine/aromatherapy/aromatherapy-eucalyptus.htm (accessed 6 Jun 2013).

• Medline Plus. "Eucalyptus: MedlinePlus Supplements." 2012. http://www.nlm.nih.gov/medlineplus/druginfo/natural/700.html (accessed 6 Jun 2013).

• RxList. "Eucalyptus Effectiveness, Safety, and Drug Interactions on RxList." 2013. http://www.rxlist.com/eucalyptus/supplements.htm (accessed 6 Jun 2013).

• University of Maryland Medical Center. "Eucalyptus." 2012. http://www.umm.edu/altmed/articles/eucalyptus-000241.htm (accessed 6 Jun 2013).

• WebMD. "EUCALYPTUS: Uses, Side Effects, Interactions and Warnings - WebMD." 2009. http://www.webmd.com/vitamins-supplements/ingredientmono-700-EUCALYPTUS.aspx?activeIngredientId=700&activeIngredientName =EUCALYPTUS (accessed 6 Jun 2013).

EVENING PRIMROSE- The evening primrose is a flowering plant known by its scientific name Oenothera biennis or its other common names, evening star, German rampion, hogweed, sun drop, King's cure-all, and fever plant. The name comes from the plant's ability to bloom visibly fast during the evening.

Growing evening primrose

The evening primrose is a local plant of eastern and central North America up to regions that enjoy temperate and subtropical climate. It has yellow, four-petal flowers that are surrounded by narrow, lance-like leaves. The flowers bloom from late spring to late summer. It has a fruit that looks like a capsule and contains multiple slender seeds.

Once planted, a circle of leaves will grow after a year. Eventually, the leaves will grow alternatingly on both sides of the stem. The flowers will bloom usually from June to September, more visibly after sunset and even on cloudy days on its second year.

Benefits of evening primrose

The beauty of the evening primrose is undeniable but the essential fatty acids derived from its seeds are most prized for the numerous health benefits it can provide. It can relieve pains of premenstrual stress syndrome. It can also keep the skin supple and clear. When used as a poultice, it can heal bruises and hasten wound healing.

The Native American Indians have been using its leaves, roots and seed pods for conditions such as haemorrhoids and other skin problems. People take evening primrose oil for rheumatoid arthritis, psoriasis, eczema, and breast pain experienced during menstruation. Since it has oestrogen-like properties, evening primrose oil can also prevent hypertension during pregnancy, starting and keeping labour short, relieve symptoms of menopause, and as an adjunct to endometriosis therapy. In fact, the GLA content of EPO is said to prevent male impotence by promoting blood flow and female infertility by improving uterine functions.

Manufacturers of evening primrose oil (EPO) have claimed it can help Raynaud's syndrome, multiple sclerosis, Sjogren's syndrome, Alzheimer's diseases, schizophrenia, and alcoholism. Nerve related conditions such as dyspraxia in children, nerve related damage caused by diabetes, relief from itching caused by neurodermatitis, and attention deficit-hyperactivity disorder (ADHD). This is due to the GLA's ability to produce prostaglandin E which helps prevent depression and seizures. Even circulatory problems such as leg pain caused by blocked blood vessels, heart disease, and high cholesterol use EPO.

What to look out for

Some people will use evening primrose oil without any side effects. Complications that can be experienced when taking in the oil are headache, stomach upset, diarrhea, and transient bouts of nausea. Since it has characteristics similar to oestrogen, breastfeeding and pregnant women should not use this supplement.

Medications may also complicate the use of evening primrose oil. Those taking blood thinning medications such as antiplatelet and anticoagulants become more at risk for bleeding. People diagnosed with schizophrenia, depression, and other psychotic conditions will have an increased risk for seizures as well as intense episodes of nausea and vomiting, especially if they're taking phenothiazines. It can also cause an extreme drop of blood pressure in people taking antihypertensive medications. Herbs such as danshen, garlic, and ginger might also interact with EPO and cause bleeding.

Avoid using evening primrose oil a fortnight before any scheduled surgery or dental procedure that involves the use of anaesthesia. The oil will cause seizures similar to those taking phenothiazines.

How to use evening primrose

The young leaves of evening primrose are highly edible and can be cooked as a vegetable in dishes and salads. The gamma-linolenic acid content is found in small amounts in a variety of food sources but it is more concentrated in evening primrose and borage. The

Native Americans have used this wildflower as food and medicine. European settlers brought some roots back to England and Germany where it has been consumed as food.

EPO is sold as skin creams or encapsulated oil in airtight, light-resistant containers. Standard supplements will contain eight per cent gamma-linolenic acid (GLA). These Although there is no standard dose for evening primrose oil, a dose that has been used in a study that shows EPO can relieve breast pain is about three to four grams a day. For other indications, adults can take about two to eight grams of eight per cent GLA per day. In studying the effects of evening primrose oil on eczema, the dose found most effective is four to eight grams daily in divided doses. Studies involving children on the effects of evening primrose oil on their skin have used three grams of EPO in divided doses per day but no more than 0.5 gram per kilogram of their body weight.

Studies on evening primrose

The seeds of the evening primrose contain about seven to 10 per cent of gamma-linolenic acid, an essential fatty acid. It is rich in omega-6 which is necessary for good health. Nonetheless, results of such studies on this plant have been conflicting. Some studies done are often small and badly designed.

Reviews on the available scientific data for evening primrose oil's beneficial effects that claim to relieve the discomfort of premenstrual syndrome during menstruation, ADHD, and hot flashes during menopause are not that effective.

What some research has shown is that evening primrose oil may be beneficial for eczema or atopic dermatitis. The gamma-linolenic acid content in the oils may have some benefit for those suffering from joint pains. Still, the use of EPO may be effective for breast pain, although not for a long time, and osteoporosis when combined with calcium minerals and omega-3 rich fish oils. However, more trials and research are needed to prove this.

According to experts, there are other herbs more effective for such indications. Chaste tree or vitamin B6 with calcium and magnesium are believed to be more effective than EPO when relieving breast pain. There is not enough evidence that evening primrose oil has any value when used as a complementary treatment for certain cancers. The same is true for all the other claims that manufacturers of evening primrose oil.

References:

• Mayo Clinic. "Evening primrose oil (Oenothera biennis L.) - MayoClinic.com." 2012.
http://www.mayoclinic.com/health/evening-primrose-oil/NS_patient-primrose (accessed 06 Jun 2013).

• Medicine Net. "EVENING PRIMROSE OIL - ORAL side effects, medical uses, and drug interactions.." 2013.

http://www.medicinenet.com/evening_primrose_oil-oral/article.htm (accessed 06 Jun 2013).

• Medline Plus. "Evening primrose oil: MedlinePlus Supplements." 2008. http://www.nlm.nih.gov/medlineplus/druginfo/natural/1006.html (accessed 06 Jun 2013).

• University of Maryland Medical Center. "Evening primrose oil." 2012. http://www.umm.edu/altmed/articles/evening-primrose-000242.htm (accessed 06 Jun 2013).

WebMD. "Evening Primrose Oil: Uses and Risks." 2012. http://www.webmd.com/vitamins-and-supplements/evening-primrose-oil-uses-and-risks (accessed 06 Jun 2013).

FENNEL- Fennel is an aromatic herb with small, yellow flowers and feathery leaves local to Mediterranean shores. Its scientific name is Foeniculum vulgare and also known by its common names carosella, fenouil, finnochio, hinojo, sanuf, shatapushpha, and xiao hui xiang. It has also been a popular mainstay in the kitchen. The name came from "fenyl" in Middle English and comes from the Latin word,"faenum" or hay.

Growing fennel

The herb has been mentioned in Greek mythology where Prometheus stole fire from the gods using fennel stalks. The hollow stems are erect and green, with threadlike leaves that grow up to more than a foot long. The yellow flowers form a bell-like formation. The most important part of the herb is the fruit that appears to be a grooved seed that can grow to about a third of an inch.

This Mediterranean herb has been naturalised in other countries such as Northern Europe, the United States, southern Canada, Asia, and some parts of Australia. As of 2008, India is the major producer of fennel. Fennel will grow anywhere and will last for years. Those who cultivate the herb sow it from seeds, usually in April. It prefers a lot of sun and will not need heavy use of fertilisers in order to survive. Nonetheless, heavily manured soil will yield a lot of fruits. More than two kilograms of seeds are enough to cover an acre, about 15 inches apart, sewn lightly and eventually transplanted when mature..

Like herbs that are valuable in healing and in the kitchen, fennel has been widely cultivated for its edible, flavourful leaves and its aromatic, tasty fruits. Florence fennel is a variety of the common fennel as it has a bulbous leaf base. It has a mild, sweet flavour and highly aromatic.

Benefits of fennel

Indians and Romans have eaten sweetened fennel seeds to improve eyesight. The fennel root's extracts are treated as eye tonics to clear cloudy vision. The Fennel herb has in past and currently been utilized to improve milk flow in breastfeeding mothers, although there is no direct evidence for it. Women have used fennel to promote menstruation, ease up labour, and improve sex drive. Manufacturers of breast enhancement products have included fennel as one of their ingredients.

Fennel is rich in phytonutrients that gives it strong antioxidant properties. Surprisingly, it is rich in vitamin C which neutralises free radicals that can cause cell damage and provide a natural antimicrobial minus the bacterial resistance. It has folate which keeps homocysteine, a chemical that might ravage blood vessels, in check.

This spice is employed for a variety of digestive conditions such as heartburn, gas, bloating, and loss of appetite. It has also been utilised for infections of the upper respiratory tract, coughs, bronchitis, cholera, back pain, and to stop bedwetting. A poultice of fennel powder is believed to heal snakebites. Ingesting fennel is supposedly an antidote for poisoning.

What to look out for

When used short term, fennel is generally safe. However, since it has oestrogen-like effects, women who have certain cancers and gynaecological conditions, such as endometriosis and uterine fibroids, should steer clear from fennel. People with allergies to celery, carrots, mugwort, and other similar plants will tend to develop an allergy to fennel.

Fennel use may also interact with certain medications. Drugs such as birth control pills, ciprofloxacin, oestrogen-containing medications, and tamoxifen might be less effective than usual. It affects most medications that needs to be metabolised by the liver and those that contain or counteract oestrogen in the body.

How to use fennel

Fennel and anise are prime ingredients in making absinthe. The bulbs of the cultivated Florence fennel are eaten raw or cooked like a vegetable. Aside from the bulb, the leaves and the seeds are part of many culinary traditions (think Indian, Pakistan, Afghan, Iranian, Chinese, Spanish, and Middle Eastern) all over the world. The small flowers (also known as fennel pollen in the US) are very expensive and the most potent. The seeds are often used as spice, with green seeds packing in the most flavour. Leaves are treated similar to dill and eaten in soups, sauces, and salads.

The essence of fennel has been used as an herbal medication for dysmenorrhea, although mefenamic acid is more potent. It has also been utilized to relieve flatulence in both humans and animals. When mixed with syrup, it can be given to colicky children. The syrup has been given for chronic coughs.

When given for its stimulant and carminative properties, a dose of five to seven grams for the seed and 0.1 to 0.6 millilitres for the oil are given daily in divided doses.

Studies on fennel

The seeds of the fennel herb holds about three to six per cent of necessary oil along with about 20 per cent of fixed oil made up of oleic acid, petroselinic acid, as well as vitamin E. The essential oil contains 90 per cent anethole, 20 per cent fenchone, and the remaining a mix of camphor, limonene, pinene and other compounds such as hydroxybenzoic acid and caffeic acid. Seeds and leaves of the fennel are rich in quercetin and kaempferol.

Anethole is a major aromatic chemical found in anise and star anise, but more pronounced in fennel seeds. This compound shuts down the biochemical signals that release tumor necrosis factor (TNF) which prevents gene alteration and inflammation in the body. It is also rich in substances such as estragole that have an oestrogen-like effect. Fennel is believed to work by relaxing the large intestine and lessen the secretions of the respiratory tract.

There are animal studies that have shown fennel extracts' ability to treat glaucoma. In 2007, fennel has been listed as one of the potential herbal antihypertensive because of its diuretic effect.

There are insufficient studies that show fennel extracts are effective for indigestion, bronchitis, flatulence, and infections of the upper respiratory tract.

There is a study that has shown fennel oil being genotoxic to the DNA of Bacillus subtilis. The estragole content in the volatile oil has triggered tumour formation in test animals.

References:

- Botanical.com. "A Modern Herbal | Fennel." 1995. http://botanical.com/botanical/mgmh/f/fennel01.html (accessed 07 Jun 2013).

- Drugs.com. "Fennel professional information from Drugs.com." 2009. http://www.drugs.com/npp/fennel.html (accessed 07 Jun 2013).

- Medicine Net. "Fennel Information | Evidenced-Based Supplement Guide on MedicineNet.com." 2013. http://www.medicinenet.com/fennel/supplements-vitamins.htm (accessed 07 Jun 2013).

- RxList. "Fennel Effectiveness, Safety, and Drug Interactions on RxList." 2013. http://www.rxlist.com/fennel/supplements.htm (accessed 07 Jun 2013).

- WebMD. "FENNEL: Uses, Side Effects, Interactions and Warnings - WebMD." 2009. http://www.webmd.com/vitamins-supplements/ingredientmono-311-FENNEL.aspx?activeIngredientId=311&activeIngredientName=FENNEL (accessed 07 Jun 2013).

FENUGREEK- Fenugreek is an herb that is highly valued for its seeds. Its scientific name is Trigonella foenugraecum but it is also known as bird's foot, Greek clover, alholva, bockshornklee, methika, h ulu ba, and senegrain. It smells and tastes like maple syrup which makes it a valuable ingredient in spice blends and flavouring to imitate maple syrup.

Growing fenugreek

As one of mankind's oldest surviving medicinal plants, Assyrians have been cultivating it 3000 years ago. The plant is related to the beans and legumes but somewhat hairy. Its slender stems carry egg-shaped leaves while root appears to have an extensive network underground. The flowers often appear white or pale yellow. Its seed pods are slender with beak-like tips which might contain 10 to 20 seeds. Even when planted on the ground, fenugreek will emit a spicy odour that adheres to the hands tenaciously. It tastes somewhat aromatic and bittersweet.

Fenugreek is relatively native to Syrian, Lebanon, India, China, and some parts of southeast Europe. However, it has been cultivated in countries such as France, Argentina, Egypt, and Ethiopia. The Romans have imported the herb from Greece because it was used as fodder for their cattle. People in the Middle East, India and some parts of the Far East have used it as nutritious herb in their diets where it is often incorporated as an ingredient in curry powder.

Fenugreek grows from seeds and is often treated with Azospirillum before being sown in June and October. The plant grows best in rich, loamy soil that has ample drainage. Commercial cultivation often sows 12 kilos of seeds per hectare. The sown plants are often thinned, 25 days after, with the harvest being consumed as greens. About three months need to pass before the grains can be harvested.

Benefits of fenugreek

There are many health benefits attributed to fenugreek. It has been utilised for problems of the skin, digestive tract, urinary tract, upper respiratory tract, and circulatory system. It can also benefit people with diabetes, address male problems and promote milk flow in breastfeeding women.

What to look out for

When taken in amounts found in food, fenugreek is expected to produce no untoward effects. Larger amounts consumed when taken as medicine, there are some side effects that might be experienced. Diarrhea, gastric discomfort, bloating, flatulence, and that characteristic maple syrup smell in the urine. Aside from these, expect fenugreek to cause some nasal congestion, coughing, gasping, and some allergic reactions in people sensitive to fenugreek.

Since fenugreek has some oestrogen-like properties, it is unsafe for pregnant women to consume more than what is usually found in food. It can cause premature contractions. Women who have taken fenugreek before giving birth might cause the infant to emit an unusual maple syrup body odour that could be mistaken for a type of ketoaciduria, an autosomal disorder.

Breastfeeding women who rely on fenugreek to jumpstart their milk flow should be wary that there is no available scientific data that proves fenugreek is safe to use when breastfeeding. What is known is that fenugreek is dangerous for children as they might faint or develop that maple syrup body odour.

As fenugreek can lower blood sugar drastically, especially in people with diabetes, make sure that the levels of blood glucose is monitored regularly. It can also interact with the maintenance medications they take. Either the dose needs to be adjusted or rigid monitoring be done when using fenugreek. Some anti-diabetic drugs that will interact with fenugreek are glimepride, pioglitazone, insulin, tolbutamide, chlorpropamide, and others.

Fenugreek can also interact with drugs that are blood thinners. It might slow down blood clotting which means there is an increased risk for bruising and bleeding. Some medications to watch out for are warfarin, aspirin, clopidogrel, dalteparin, and other similar drugs.

How to use fenugreek

Fenugreek is used at times as a poultice to treat local pain and swelling. The seeds may be ground or whole, wrapped in cloth and warmed before being applied in a specific sore or inflamed part. This makes the herb valuable for muscle and joint pains, swollen lymph nodes, gout, ulcers on the skin, wounds, and eczema.

There is no standard dosing for fenugreek nor is there any regulating body that can assess products containing fenugreek for their purity and quality. When using fenugreek, use it as directed or consult your health professional before using. Never use different forms of fenugreek containing products at the same time to prevent overdose.

The United States and Europe have long waived fenugreek from its armada of herbal medications. On the other hand, people in India have continued treating the plant both as an herbal medication and nourishing food.

Fenugreek is eaten as a vegetable in India. It can be used raw or roasted to flavour mango chutney. Although the seeds are highly prized, the sprouts are often eaten uncooked in salads.

Studies on fenugreek

Fenugreek has shown potential as an anti-diabetic medication. When consumed with food during meals, people affected with either Type I or Type II diabetes have remarkably lower blood glucose than usual. Experts believe that fenugreek can slow down how the body takes in sugar in the stomach and helps stimulate insulin production. It can be through fenugreek's 4-hydroxyleucine content which stimulates insulin production when blood sugar spikes.

The seeds of the fenugreek contain diosgenin, which can be used to manufacture progesterone that gives the herb an ability to affect gynaecological conditions. Trigonelle, another component of the seed, is changed into niacin when the seeds are roasted.

Although there is conflicting scientific data on fenugreek's ability to control bad cholesterol, what is known in preliminary research is that it can lower triglycerides in people with Type II diabetes.

In spite of these folk remedies, there is not enough scientific evidence to prove whether it is really effective. Conditions such as poor sexual performance, baldness, and other conditions attributed to benefit from the use of fenugreek have yet to provide enough evidence to show their effectiveness in general.

@Arthur Bramble@

References:

•   UCLA Louise M Darling Biomedical Library. "Medicinal Spices Exhibit - UCLA Biomedical Library: History & Special Collections." 2002. http://unitproj.library.ucla.edu/biomed/spice/index.cfm?displayID=13 (accessed 07 Jun 2013).

•   RxList. "Fenugreek Effectiveness, Safety, and Drug Interactions on RxList." 2013. http://www.rxlist.com/fenugreek/supplements.htm (accessed 07 Jun 2013).

•   National Center for Complementary and Alternative Medicine (NCCAM). "Fenugreek | NCCAM." 2007. http://nccam.nih.gov/health/fenugreek (accessed 07 Jun 2013).

•   Drugs.com. "Fenugreek medical facts from Drugs.com." 2010. http://www.drugs.com/mtm/fenugreek.html (accessed 07 Jun 2013).

WebMD. "FENUGREEK: Uses, Side Effects, Interactions and Warnings - WebMD." 2009. http://www.webmd.com/vitamins-supplements/ingredientmono-733-FENUGREEK.aspx?activeIngredientId=733&activeIngredientName=FENUGREEK (accessed 07 Jun 2013).

FEVERFEW- Feverfew is a very old medicinal herb that has been used initially as an anti-inflammatory and as a major treatment for fever. The name comes from the Latin word "febrifugia" which means fever reducer. Its scientific name is Tanacetum parthenium and is a relative of daisies. It is known by its common name altamisa, featherfoil, Santa Maria, flirtroot, and wild quinine. At present, people use feverfew to relieve migraine headaches.

Growing feverfew

The feverfew plant is local to South Eastern Europe (specifically, the Balkan peninsula) but it has spread throughout Europe, North America, and Australia. It has been used by Greek physician Dioscorides similar to how aspirin is used today. The Kallaway Indians have used it for colic, kidney pain, and morning sickness. Danish medicine has used it as a natural remedy for epilepsy.

Feverfew is a short, bushy perennial that grows up to a metre in height. The plant blooms from July to October and will often give off a heavy bitter odour. The yellow-green leaves are arranged alternately and have small, yellow flowers that look like daisies and chamomiles which can lead to confusion.

Benefits of feverfew

Although popularly used as an herbal treatment for migraines, feverfew offers a wide array of health benefits. Aside from lowering temperatures in fevers, it can regulate irregular menstruation, psoriasis, arthritis, ringing in the ears, dizziness, and even nausea. Some people believe that feverfew can help with infertility or help prevent miscarriage, anaemia, common colds, liver problems, muscle strains, and oedema of the extremities. Locally, it can be applied on gums for toothaches or on the skin as an antiseptic. It has been used for opium overdose.

What to look out for

When used short term or not more than four months, feverfew is safe. However that does not mean that one can be spared from the side effects of feverfew in the system. Side effects often involve gastrointestinal upset, heartburn, irregular bowel movements, gas, and nausea. Other people have reported experiencing anxiety, vertigo, headache, difficulty sleeping, stiffness of joints, rash, irregular heartbeat and weight gain. However, these side effects cannot be fully blamed on feverfew as there is a high probability that the supplement may be adulterated.

Pills made of feverfew should be swallowed whole instead of being chewed down. Chewing feverfew supplements might cause mouth sores, swollen mouth cavity, and a temporary loss of taste. Women who are pregnant or breastfeeding as there aren't any studies that show feverfew is safe for such conditions. Some research has shown feverfew can stimulate premature contractions and worse, miscarriage. People allergic to ragweed and other related plants such as chrysanthemums, marigolds, and daisies might also be allergic to feverfew. It might also thin the blood so people should stop using it a fortnight before a scheduled surgery.

Medications that are metabolised in the liver will interact with the use of feverfew. These drugs' effects might be further potentiated but it also carries with it a higher risk of experiencing their side effects. Some medications to watch out for are the non-steroidal anti-inflammatory drugs (NSAIDs) such as ibuprofen, piroxicam, aspirin, as well as glipizide, losartan, lovastatin, itraconazole, and enoxaparin.

How to use feverfew

Feverfew supplements are sold as fresh, freeze dried or dried. These are often available in capsules, tablets, or liquid extract and should contain about 0.2 per cent of parthenolide but some formulations can contain as much as 0.7 per cent of parthenolide.

There are no standard doses for feverfew. What has been used in scientific research that has shown promise to prevent migraine headaches is 50 to 100 milligrams of feverfew extracts in divided doses every day. Alternatively, some people are given 100 to 300 milligrams of feverfew extracts containing 0.2 to 0.4 per cent of parthenolide in divided doses of up to every six hours. Carbon dioxide extracted feverfew extracts are taken at 6.25 milligrams every eight hours for up to four months.

People suffering from rheumatoid arthritis are given three to six millilitres of 1:1 feverfew fluid extract twice a day or about three to six millilitres of 1:5 feverfew tinctures every 12 hours.

Studies on feverfew

Pathenolide and other chemicals found in feverfew leaves might lower the incidence of suffering a migraine headache. Researchers believe that this compound can relieve the spasms of the smooth muscles. There is some evidence that feverfew can lower the frequency of attacks and decrease the discomfort, nausea and vomiting as well as increased tolerance to light and noise. The herb is more potent on people who are more prone to suffer the attacks. Another study reveals that there is no other effect except as placebo. A critical review showed that the effects varied with the types of products being used. The Canadian government allowed manufacturers that have 0.2 per cent of the parthenolide so that the latter can claim it can prevent migraines.

In the 1980's, feverfew became a popular herbal treatment for migraine headaches in Great Britain. On a survey conducted on 270 people using the herb, about 70 per cent of them agree that they experienced relief from migraine headaches after consuming two or three fresh leaves daily. Another study combined feverfew with willow where participants took the combination every 12 hours for about three months. Their migraine headaches' duration and pain were more bearable than usual.

Using feverfew for rheumatoid arthritis might actually be ineffective. According to initial reports, taking feverfew orally does not improve the symptoms of pain or swelling associated with this type of arthritis. However, human studies have shown it to be no better than the placebo. Other conditions that claim that feverfew can cure or relieve their condition might need more evidence and scientific data so that they can be under feverfew's indication.

There are anecdotal evidence that supports the use of feverfew for fever, irregular menstruation, psoriasis, asthma, earache, and the common cold. However, there is very little evidence that can be systematically verified for its use to be endorsed by the scientific community.

References:

• National Center for Complementary and Alternative Medicine (NCCAM). "Feverfew | NCCAM." 2006. http://nccam.nih.gov/health/feverfew (accessed 08 Jun 2013).

• RxList. "Feverfew Effectiveness, Safety, and Drug Interactions on RxList." 2013. http://www.rxlist.com/feverfew/supplements.htm (accessed 08 Jun 2013).

- University of Maryland Medical Center. "Feverfew." 2012. http://www.umm.edu/altmed/articles/feverfew-000243.htm (accessed 08 Jun 2013).

- WebMD. "FEVERFEW: Uses, Side Effects, Interactions and Warnings - WebMD." 2009. http://www.webmd.com/vitamins-supplements/ingredientmono-933-FEVERFEW.aspx?activeIngredientId=933&activeIngredientName=FEVERFEW (accessed 08 Jun 2013).

- Drugs.com. "Feverfew professional information from Drugs.com." 2009. http://www.drugs.com/npp/feverfew.html (accessed 08 Jun 2013).

GARLIC- Garlic is an herb that has been made famous by Hollywood's vampire movies, praised by celebrity chefs, and touted by herbalists as a miracle cure for a variety of medical conditions. Its scientific name is Allium sativum and a close relative of another kitchen mainstay, the onion. It's a bulb made up of separate cloves. Garlic is also known as rustic treacle and stinking rose. In other countries, it's known as ajo in Spanish, ail in French, and da suan in Mandarin.

Growing garlic

Botanists have traced the origin of the garlic to Central and South West Asia as a common weed. Planting it for personal consumption is made possible by sowing separate cloves in temperate climates. It should be at least four inches deep with minimal spaces between. These grow well in loose, dry soils that are well-drained and rich with organic material.

Benefits of garlic

Humans have long used garlic for thousands of years. One of the most popular uses of garlic is rubbing it on snake bites. Its oil is believed to dissolve the venom in the lymphatic system. Traditional herbal treatments also involve rubbing in garlic on skin disorders and on the scalp where there is hair thinning. Another folk remedy for garlic involves applying it directly on acne outbreaks. It has been used as a spice to prevent food poisoning. During the previous World Wars, soldiers have used garlic to prevent gangrene when antibiotics are not available.

Garlic is used as a dietary supplement to keep levels of bad cholesterol in check, especially in people prone to cardiovascular diseases and high blood pressure. People with diabetes, osteoarthritis, hay fever, pre-eclampsia, and upper respiratory tract infections also use garlic. Its oil can also be applied to fungal infections, such as athlete's foot or ringworm. Some people also use the oil to treat calluses and warts. Consuming garlic regularly reduces tick bites while rubbing it on will repel mosquitoes.

What to look out for

Although garlic is generally safe for most people, it can present certain side effects. Consuming raw cloves will often bring about body odour, increase stomach upset, and allergies. It can decrease clotting factors in the blood that makes one prone to bleeding. When used on the skin, its sulphur content may cause a burning sensation.

Treating with garlic may also interfere on how certain medications act on the body. Potentially deadly combinations involve isoniazid, group of antiviral medications against Human Immunodeficiency Virus (HIV), and saquinavir Garlic can either prevent the drug's absorption, as in the case of isoniazid, or hasten the breakdown of medication inside the body, such as saquinavir and other anti-retrovirals for HIV.

Use garlic with caution when taking pills for contraception, cyclosporine, blood thinners, and those that pass through the liver to be metabolised. Birth control pills, lovastatin, ketoconazole, fexofenadine, triazolam, and cyclosporine may not be effective when taken with garlic because the latter helps the body break them down faster and rendering them ineffective. Paracetamol, theophylline, and some anaesthetics might accumulate in the body and cause toxic side effects. Blood thinners might be more potent than usual and increase the risk for bleeding.

How to use garlic

Garlic can be eaten raw or cooked. Some manufacturers have processed garlic into tablets and capsules while others extract the oil into soft gel capsules. Every garlic preparation's potency depends on the amount of allicin, garlic's active ingredient. A milligram of allicin is said to be equal to 15 units of penicillin. One clove of fresh garlic daily can be used to control hypertension. For those who find fresh garlic unpalatable, commercially made extracts containing 1.3 per cent of allin can be used. About 600 milligrams to 1.2 grams of garlic extract may be divided and taken thrice a day.

In the kitchen, garlic has always been a mainstay in Mediterranean cuisine. Aside from being an antidote to poisons by the Romans, it has been employed by the Spanish as a preservative for food. Ancient Egyptians believed it enhances their strength and endurance. Asians have used it both as a spice and condiment.

Garlic is also potent when used locally. For skin infections, about 0.4 to 1.0 per cent of ajoene gel may be applied twice daily. For those who want to use garlic as is, crushing raw garlic and allow it to set for seven 14 minutes, will allow a sufficient increase in allicin and kill Staphylococci and Streptococci bacteria, even those who have gone resistant.

Studies on garlic

According to some studies, consuming garlic has shown potential in lowering unwanted cholesterol, slow down the hardening of blood vessels, lower blood pressure, and lessen the tendency to have certain types of cancer. The diallyl sulphide in garlic is a potent constituent that prevents disease development. This has helped many people improve after taking garlic supplements regularly.

Colon, rectal, and stomach cancer are some types of cancers that is said to be prevented with regular use of garlic. Scientists discovered that people who consume large amounts of garlic and their relatives, such as onions or scallions, have lower risk for cancers that affect the gastrointestinal tract. Experts attribute this to garlic's ability to prevent carcinogens, such as nitrosamines, from building up in the digestive system.

More evidence has yet to be provided for people who claim it can be useful for conditions of the prostate. Some preliminary results have shown consuming raw garlic may relieve symptoms of benign prostatic hyperplasia (BPH). In China, men who consume a clove a clove a day slash their risk of developing prostate cancer.

Studies funded by the National Center for Complementary and Alternative Medicine (NCCAM) show very little significant benefit. What is certain, according to the NCCAM, is that garlic has an effect on other medications since it can affect liver function and blood circulation. A study funded by the National Sciences and Engineering Research Council of Canada (NSERC) and the Ontario Ministry of Innovation scrutinized allicin as a potent antioxidant. The results showed that allicin needs to decompose to release sulfenic acid, which acts as a potent antioxidant to the body's free radicals.

References:

• Medline plus. "Garlic." 2011. http://www.nlm.nih.gov/medlineplus/druginfo/natural/300.html (accessed 18 May 2013).

• National Center for Complementary and Alternative Medicine (NCCAM). "Herbs at a Glance: Garlic." 2006. http://nccam.nih.gov/health/garlic/ataglance.htm (accessed 18 May 2013).

- University of Maryland Medical Center. "Garlic." 2011. http://www.umm.edu/altmed/articles/garlic-000245.htm (accessed 18 May 2013).

- WebMD. "GARLIC." 2009. http://www.webmd.com/vitamins-supplements/ingredientmono-300-GARLIC.aspx?activeIngredientId=300&activeIngredientName=GARLIC (accessed 18 May 2013).

- The New York Times. "After 4,000 Years, Medical Science Considers Garlic." 1990. http://www.nytimes.com/1990/09/04/science/after-4000-years-medical-science-considers-garlic.html?pagewanted=all&src=pm (accessed 18 May 2013).

GINGER-   Ginger is an herb that is valued for its rhizome that is used as a spice and herbal medicine. Its scientific name is Zingiber officinale and has been known by other names such as gan jiang, imber, kankyo, nagara, shokyp, and sunthi, depending on location.

Growing ginger

Ginger has been a part of Asian, Indian, and Arabic herbal medicine since ancient times. This potent thizome is a native of Asia and has been used as a kitchen spice for over four millennia.

The knobby, thick, beige underground stem of the ginger is the most prized part of the plant. The stem that grows above ground will grow up to a feet high with long, slender, ridged green leaves and will sport mildly fragrant yellowish-green or white flowers.

Benefits of ginger

The rhizomes of the ginger are given for many conditions related to digestion. Nausea from motion sickness, morning sickness, colic, gas, nausea due to cancer chemotherapy, and loss of appetite can benefit from the use of ginger. It can also relieve pain caused by arthritis, muscle strain, dysmenorrhea, chest pain, lumbago, and stomach pain. If applied on the skin, ginger extracts can treat burns and as spot on treatment for pain.

What to look out for

Ginger is very safe for most people but some people might experience mild side effects such as heartburn, diarrhoea, and some discomfort in the stomach. Women have reported profuse menstrual bleeding when taking ginger.

Using ginger during pregnancy is somewhat debatable. There is some apprehension that ginger might affect the foetuses' sex hormones.

The report of miscarriage on the third month of pregnancy is alarming. However, there some data that shows that the risk of premature labour, low birth weight or malformations since birth on women using ginger is not that abnormally high when compared to the usual one to three per cent to those who do not use ginger.

What is a major concern is the risk for uncontrolled bleeding so it is best to stop using ginger before the last trimester.

Since ginger is a natural blood thinner, it can interact with anticoagulants and antiplatelet drugs. This means there is an increased chance of uncontrolled bleeding or bruising. It may interact with herbs that are natural blood thinners such as angelica, clove, garlic, ginkgo, ginseng, turmeric, and other herbs that have similar properties.

There is no data that shows ginger is safe to use during breastfeeding. Stay safe and avoid it. Ginger can lower blood sugar so monitor its levels regularly or have your physician adjust the dosage of anti-diabetic medications. Some medications to watch out for are glimepride, pioglitazone, insulin, chlorpropamide, and other similar drugs.

Too much ginger, on the other hand, might worsen some heart conditions. It can reduce blood pressure so low that it might starve the heart of the much needed circulation it needs. It can also interact with antihypertensive medications that block calcium that makes the blood pressure drop dangerously low. Drugs to watch out for are nifedipine, verapamil, diltiazem, and other similar medications.

How to use ginger

Although there are no standard doses for ginger as a herbal remedy. However, there are doses that have been effective for certain indications. For women suffering from morning sickness, take 250 milligrams of ginger extract every six hours. For those who want to keep nausea and vomiting after surgery, one to two grams of powdered ginger may be given, an hour before anaesthesia is given. For people suffering from arthritis, ginger extract doses are highly variable, depending on the packaging instructions. It can range from twice to four times daily.

Ginger may be used fresh, dried and ground into fine powder, as juice, or oil. It should contain four per cent of its volatile oils or about five per cent of pungent chemicals that includes both shogaol and gingerol. As a general rule, do not take more than four grams a day. Pregnant women should consume less than a gram daily.

Studies on ginger

Ginger may contain chemicals that can reduce queasiness and soreness that acts locally in the stomach and the intestines. Some of these chemicals act on the nervous system to control bouts of nausea. Its active component are pungent compounds known as gingerols and shogaols.

Ginger has shown promise in preventing nausea and vomiting after surgery and in averting morning sickness. According to some clinical trials, a gram of ginger an hour before surgery will keep nausea and vomiting at bay by 38 per cent for about 24 hours after surgery. However, it cannot stop bouts of vomiting and nausea three to six hours post-surgery. On the other hand, some pregnant women seem to benefit from taking ginger or any of its extracts to keep everything in. Despite the data on hand, researchers still recommend consulting a health professional about possible risks.

There are some data that demonstrated ginger's effectiveness in controlling pain.

There are some studies that have shown ginger can lessen the discomfort caused by menstruation in some women.

In fact, there is a specific ginger extract that is taken three days upon the start of menstruation which lowers the incidence of menstrual pain by 62 per cent, comparable to the benefits gained from using ibuprofen or mefenamic acid.

Arthritic pain, on the other hand, is said to be moderately reduced on people affected with osteoarthritis.

There are specific ginger extracts from different manufacturers that provided data that it almost comparable to ibuprofen in relieving pain.

A separate study showed that ginger combined with glucosamine worked just as well as diclofenac and glucosamine. There are preliminary evidence that ginger extracts can help lower joint pain in rheumatoid arthritis.

What is established right now is that ginger might not be effective in preventing vertigo. There are anecdotal evidence that some people actually feel better when taking ginger before they travel. However, there is no data that the herb actually does that.

There is insufficient evidence that ginger is effective for improving appetite, colds, and flu.

References:

- Discovery Health. ""Ginger Health Benefits"." 2009. http://health.howstuffworks.com/wellness/natural-medicine/alternative/ginger-fight-cancer1.htm (accessed 08 Jun 2013).

- Medline Plus. "Ginger: MedlinePlus Supplements." 2012. http://www.nlm.nih.gov/medlineplus/druginfo/natural/961.html (accessed 08 Jun 2013).

- National Center for Complementary and Alternative Medicine (NCCAM). "Ginger | NCCAM." 2006. http://nccam.nih.gov/health/ginger (accessed 08 Jun 2013).

- University of Maryland Medical Center. "Ginger." 2012. http://www.umm.edu/altmed/articles/ginger-000246.htm (accessed 08 Jun 2013).

- WebMD. "GINGER: Uses, Side Effects, Interactions and Warnings - WebMD." 2009. http://www.webmd.com/vitamins-supplements/ingredientmono-961-GINGER.aspx?activeIngredientId=961&activeIngredientName=GINGER (accessed 08 Jun 2013).

GINKGO (GINKGO BILOBA) - Ginkgo is an ancient tree whose leaves are extracted for the medicinal benefits it provides. It's known for its scientific name Ginkgo biloba but laymen refer to it as the maidenhair tree, fossil tree, Kew tree, or Japanese silver apricot. Other people refer to it as adiantifolia, arbre du ciel, or yinshing.

Growing ginkgo

Ginkgo is a living fossil that has remained unchanged for billions of years. It is believed that the tree can live for millennia or more. The ginkgo is a native of China and is highly cultivated in Buddhist temples and Japanese gardens. These plants can adapt well even in an urban environment by tolerating pollution and small soil spaces.

Ginkgoes are large trees which can be as tall as 66 to 115 feet. It has deep roots and is highly resistant to frost and wind. When young, the tree will appear tall and slender and eventually grow gnarly as it ages. It will grow best in a sunny environment that enjoys good drainage and sufficient water. Its leaves are very unique, as it appears fan shaped that will change to yellow during autumn. Its seeds have a fleshy outmost layer that is yellowish brown, mushy, and resembles fruit. Beware though, as these contain poisonous butyric acid that will smell like vomitus when it falls from the tree. It has a hard shell inside.

Benefits of ginkgo

Ginkgo is famous for treating memory problems and for improving blood circulation in the brain. Its extracts are reputed to enhance memory, relieve headache, stop ringing in the ears, optimise focus and concentration, stabilise mood swings and augment hearing. Others have benefited from its ability to enhance blood circulation in other parts of the body such as those suffering from Raynaud's syndrome and leg pain when moving about. It has been tried for eye problems and sexual performance dysfunction. There are other claims that is said to benefit from taking ginkgo but it is mostly based on traditional use and not on scientific evidence.

What to look out for

When the seeds of the ginkgo are eaten in large amounts or for a long period of time, poisoning by methylpyridoxine may occur, especially in children. This poison is not destroyed by cooking and will cause convulsions unless treated by pyridoxine. The fleshy outer part of the seeds contains butyric acid which might cause serious allergies on contact with the skin.

When used according to label instructions, ginkgo leaf extracts are very safe. It might have some minor side effects such as gastrointestinal upset, headache, dizziness, strong heartbeat, and some rash skin rashes. There is also a risk of increased risk of bruising as ginkgo is a natural blood thinner. Children, pregnant, and infertile women should never use this herb.

How to use ginkgo

The hard nut-like insides of the seeds are highly prized delicacies in Asia. It is mixed in congee and other special dishes served only during special occasions.

For most users who have yet to use this herb, a starting dose that is lower than 120 milligrams will keep stomach discomfort away. Doses often vary based on manufacturer's instructions as there are no standard formulations for herbal supplements. The extracts are often taken by mouth.

Here are some dosages that scientific research has shown some effects on the conditions that claim to benefit from ginkgo supplements. A dose of about 120 to 240 milligrams of ginkgo leaf extract in divided doses are given for dementia. People who require better cognition require a dosage range of 120 to 600 milligrams daily. For those suffering from Raynaud's syndrome, a dose of 60 milligrams every eight hours will provide relief. Poor circulation in the lower limbs will benefit from 40 to 80 milligrams of the extract every 12 to eight hours. To avoid vertigo, a dose of 60 to 80 milligrams twice a day will suffice. Lower doses are given for premenstrual syndrome and normal tension glaucoma. From the 16th day of the menstrual cycle, a dose of 160 milligrams divided in two equal doses are taken until the fifth day of the next cycle for PMS. To relieve eye pressure, 120 milligrams in divided doses per day.

Studies on ginkgo

Ginkgo contains chemicals that improve circulation of blood and might slow down the progression of Alzheimer's disease by stopping some changes in the brain which could impede the ability to think. Its seeds are believed to contain substances that could kill bacteria and fungi.

There is some evidence that demonstrates ginkgo leaves can improve symptoms of Alzheimer's and various types of dementia. Yet there are mixed reviews as to whether the early studies were reliable. These mixed findings have yet to be decided on but actual clinical trials have proven that some symptoms have improved. It has also been able to improve short term memory of older patients with age-related memory loss and increased concentration and focus on younger people.

Clinical trials have also shown that by improving blood circulation, ginkgo leaf extracts can relieve the pain of people suffering from Raynaud's syndrome and other vascular diseases that affect the limbs. Preliminary studies have also shown that it can provide relief from breast pain and cramping associated with premenstrual syndrome as well as vertigo and motion sickness. There is also some evidence that ginkgo will benefit vision by improving pre-existing injury to those affected by glaucoma and in people with retinas damaged by diabetes. Although there have been studies that showed ginkgo's promise in helping people with age-related macular degeneration, anxiety disorders, attention deficit-hyperactivity disorder (ADHD), radiation exposure, and vitiligo, there is very little data that can be peer-reviewed to verify such claims.

Tinnitus, seasonal affective disorder, altitude sickness in climbers, and heart disease has not been effectively managed by taking ginkgo extracts. Data on ginkgo's effects on people with stroke and hearing loss are mostly conflicting. Other claims that the leaf extracts can manage high cholesterol, hardening of the arteries, certain cancers, and chronic fatigue syndrome are insufficient.

References:

•   Drugs.com. "Ginkgo medical facts from Drugs.com." 2010. http://www.drugs.com/mtm/ginkgo.html (accessed 09 Jun 2013).

•   Mayo Clinic. "Ginkgo (Ginkgo biloba) - MayoClinic.com." 2012. http://www.mayoclinic.com/health/ginkgo-biloba/NS_patient-ginkgo (accessed 09 Jun 2013).

•   MedicineNet. "GINKGO (Ginkgo biloba) - ORAL side effects, medical uses, and drug interactions.." 2013. http://www.medicinenet.com/ginkgo_ginkgo_biloba-oral/article.htm (accessed 09 Jun 2013).

•   University of Maryland Medical Center. "Ginkgo biloba." 2012. http://www.umm.edu/altmed/articles/ginkgo-biloba-000247.htm (accessed 09 Jun 2013).

WebMD. "GINKGO: Uses, Side Effects, Interactions and Warnings - WebMD." 2009. http://www.webmd.com/vitamins-supplements/ingredientmono-333-GINKGO.aspx?activeIngredientId=333&activeIngredientName=GINKGO (accessed 09 Jun 2013).

@Arthur Bramble@

GINSENG- Ginseng is a popular herbal plant that has been used as an adaptogen. There are three popular varieties used in herbal treatment: Asian ginseng, American ginseng, and Siberian ginseng. The most potent and frequently used is the Asian variety with the scientific name Panax ginseng. It is also known as Chinese, Japanese or Korean ginseng, oriental ginseng, red panax ginseng, jintsam, ren shen, and sheng shai shen. This herbal medicine has been around for two millennia and about six million Americans consume it on a regular basis.

Growing ginseng

Ginseng appears as a light tan, knobby root that has stringy shoots, sometimes taking on human form. It thrives in cooler climates and is somewhat difficult to cultivate as most ginseng grow under the canopy of trees in the forest. Roots are often left to mature for about five to ten years before it can be harvested. It can be sown from seeds that have been stored for some time or from whole roots. They need 80 per cent of shade and will survive in rich, loamy soil. It can be transferred to their permanent spot around March and April before the buds appear.

Benefits of ginseng

In general, Panax ginseng is a root that can improve mental faculties, productivity, stamina, and endurance. People take this type of ginseng to adapt to stress or as a tonic to improve over-all health. The extract can also be used to boost the performance of the immune system and to increase resistance to certain infections.

Other alternative benefits that Chinese ginseng offers are treatment for certain cancers, respiratory conditions, nervous disorders, and hormonal imbalance associated with aging. It has also been given for anaemia and other blood complaints, gastritis, and fever. Another off label uses of Asian ginseng is its ability to relieve hangovers, treat premature ejaculation and erectile dysfunction in men, and poor appetite.

What to look out for

When used for less than three months, ginseng is generally safe for most adults. However, when taken longer than that, there might be hormone-like effects that are harmful to over-all wellbeing. During the time when ginseng is taken, difficulty in sleeping is the most common complaint. Other side effects that some people might experience are irregular menstruation, fast heart rates, variable blood pressure, headache, diarrhoea, rash, and mood swings.

Pregnant women should never use ginseng because animal studies have shown that it contains a chemical that can cause birth defects in animals. Since there is no data available for nursing mothers, be on the safe side and stay clear of this herb as it is unsafe for both infants and children. There are cases where ginseng has been linked to poisoning in babies. People suffering from auto-immune diseases and organ transplants should also stay away from ginseng at it gets the immune system in hyper drive and might actually make the conditions worse. The same is true for those with hormone sensitive conditions such as endometriosis, uterine fibroids, or gynaecological cancers, since ginseng is a phytoestrogen.

Most drugs will react with red ginseng and a handful of herbs. Bitter orange and country mallow when used with ginseng can cause irregular heart rhythms which are life threatening. Herbs such as bitter melon, ginger, fenugreek, willow bark and other natural antidiabetics might cause a huge drop in levels of blood sugar. Ginseng can also interact with alcohol and caffeine. It can increase the rate of alcohol leaving your body and use up the caffeine to stimulate the nervous system causing palpitations and hypertension.

How to use ginseng

It's an enigma as to how Western medicine uses panax ginseng compared to how traditional Chinese medicine utilises the plant. For Westerners, ginseng is used as an energiser while for the Chinese; it's more of a calming, relaxing herb. Doses are often high for Chinese medicine compared to what western medicine prescribes.

Most of the doses available for ginseng are highly dependent on what is printed on their labels. However, there are standard doses that contain seven per cent of ginsenosides that have been found by scientific research to be effective for some conditions. Diabetes Type II can be controlled by taking 200 milligrams of ginseng extract daily. For those experiencing erectile dysfunction (ED), 900 milligrams every eight hours of ginseng extract are needed or a topical application of a certain cream that is applied an hour before intercourse and washed off before doing the deed.

Studies on ginseng

Panax ginseng contains a variety of active ingredients. Some of the most important chemicals are the ginsenosides (also known as panaxosides). Supplements may come as fresh roots soaked in water, alcohol or a mix or both; alternatively, it can also be in powders or capsules.

Being a potent herbal medication, manufacturers have claimed ginseng is effective for a variety of indications. However, there should be sufficient evidence based on research and clinical trials before ginseng can be proven effective. There is evidence that ingestion of Asian ginseng can actually improve cognitive skills and memory abilities, especially for people aged 38 to 66. Another potential use for ginseng is its ability to lower fasting blood sugar in people with Type II diabetes. There are studies that have also demonstrated ginseng's capacity to enhance respiration and relieve the symptoms of chronic obstructive pulmonary disease (COPD). Ginseng's effect on sexual problems in men have also been studied but with surprising results. Male impotence (ED) are improved when ginseng is taken by mouth while premature ejaculation stops when panax ginseng, along with other ingredients, are applied on the penis.

Ginseng has shown some promise in being an adjunct herbal medication for people suffering from lung infections compared to those taking antibiotics alone .Some studies exhibited that ginseng is better at preventing a cold or flu although data is currently insufficient. It is not effective for enhancing athletic performance, stabilise mood swings, or manage hot flashes during menopause. Other symptoms of menopause such as tiredness, sleeping difficulties, and depression improved when ginseng was taken orally.

References:

- Medline Plus. "Ginseng, Panax: MedlinePlus Supplements." 2012. http://www.nlm.nih.gov/medlineplus/druginfo/natural/10 00.html (accessed 09 Jun 2013).

- Medscape. "Medscape: Medscape Access." 2013. http://reference.medscape.com/drug/asian-chinese-panax-ginseng-344462 (accessed 09 Jun 2013).

- RxList. "Ginseng, Panax Effectiveness, Safety, and Drug Interactions on RxList." 2013. http://www.rxlist.com/ginseng_panax/supplements.htm (accessed 09 Jun 2013).

- University of Maryland Medical Center. "Asian ginseng." 2012. http://www.umm.edu/altmed/articles/asian-ginseng-000249.htm (accessed 09 Jun 2013).

- WebMD. "Ginseng (GINSENG, PANAX): Uses, Side Effects, Interactions and Warnings - WebMD." 2009. http://www.webmd.com/vitamins-supplements/ingredientmono-1000-Ginseng+GINSENG%2c+PANAX.aspx?activeIngredientId=1000&activeIngredientName=Ginseng+(GINSENG%2c+PANAX)&source=2&tabno=1 (accessed 09 Jun 2013).

GOLDENSEAL- Goldenseal is a plant related to the buttercup and a native of Canada.It has knobby, yellow roots that are often dried before it can be used as medicine. Its scientific name is Hydrastis Canadensis but ordinary laymen call it eye balm, golden root, ground raspberry, Indian turmeric, Racine orange, wild curcuma, or yellow puccoon.

Growing goldenseal

The goldenseal root was introduced by the Native Indian Americans to early settlers. It had been used for skin problems, digestion difficulties, and eye tonic. It has become one of the most prevalent herbal supplements in the United States alone, in spite of the lack of scientific evidence of its effects. The touted effect has almost endangered the plant from the woodlands where it once grew wild. Herbalist will often suggest using goldenseal sparingly and resort to other abundant herbals such as Oregon grape, thyme, or garlic for similar effects.

This small plant has a single hairy stem. It has sparse, lobed, and jagged leaves and small flowers that eventually bear fruit that looks like raspberry. The rhizome is bitter, often gnarled and wrinkly. It grows wild on rich, shaded soil northeast of the United States but are now cultivated in farms around the Blue Ridge Mountains, Ohio,

Kentucky, Indiana, and in Ontario, Canada. Its yellow dye had been used to colour textile and will permanently stain clothing.

Goldenseal can sprout from its rhizome. It is cut up into small pieces and planted about less than a foot apart in well-drained, humus fertilised soil that is partially shaded. Planting occurs in autumn and might take about two to three years in order to grow in its desired market size. This makes the herb very expensive in the market.

Benefits of goldenseal

There are many benefits that have been attributed to goldenseal but very few can be scientifically verified. People have sworn it's an effective eye wash for people affected with pinkeye or as cure for ringing in the ears, earache, or deafness. It has also been applied on mucous membranes affected with sores and blisters or on skin affected with rashes, ulcers, infected wounds, eczema, acne, dandruff, fungal infections, and dandruff. Aside from these, goldenseal is believed to help in urinary tract infections and in women coping with vaginal pain and soreness as well as discomfort during menstruation or bleeding after giving birth. Whooping cough, pneumonia, hay fever, stuffy nose, catching the common cold is thought to benefit from goldenseal extracts. Digestive conditions such as gastritis, peptic ulcer, inflamed intestines, irregular bowel movements; haemorrhoids, jaundice, and gas are often considered for goldenseal therapy.

What to look out for

When taken single dose, the goldenseal is relatively safe. Nevertheless, there is very little literature or reliable data that can show whether it is harmless for long term use. Do not use goldenseal when pregnant or nursing. There is compelling evidence that exposure to goldenseal or its extracts can cause brain damage in newborns. A chemical in this plant can cross the placenta and leak into breast milk.

Goldenseal extracts might actually irritate the skin, mouth, throat, and vagina when it is used topically. It can also increase the body's sensitivity to light. People with pre-existing conditions such as hypertension, liver disease, or heart conditions should discuss the possible risks of taking goldenseal with their healthcare provider. Common side effects that might be encountered when using goldenseal are nausea and drowsiness.

There are many medications that can interact with goldenseal. Drugs that need to be metabolised by liver enzymes become more potent with goldenseal since their breakdown inside the body is slowed down by the herb. Codeine, fentanyl, meperidine, metoprolol, odansetron, tramadol, ketoconazole, lovastatin, and other similar medications should be used with caution when taking goldenseal. Some drugs that work by manipulating cellular pumps might not be as effective when goldenseal is in the system. Etoposide, vincristine, indinavir, cimetidine, verapamil, corticosteroids, cisapride, cyclosporine, quinidine and other medications might become more potent and cause unnecessary exposure to side effects.

How to use goldenseal

Goldenseal supplements are sold as tablets and capsules that contain the powdered root, liquid extracts, teas, and tinctures. It often combined with another herb such as Echinacea. Sometimes, goldenseal is often used as a topical wash, mouthwash, and vaginal douche.

There is no standard dosing for goldenseal. Traditional herbalists will consider a lot of factors before giving a personalised dosage regimen to a patient. Manufacturers of goldenseal supplement will put instructions on their label which should be followed strictly.

The extreme bitterness of goldenseal has prevented many from taking it as a tea. The capsules and tinctures can mask its natural flavour. When using goldenseal tinctures, 25 to 50 drops can be used every two hours for those suffering from sore throat or infection in the digestive tract. The more frequent the dose at onset of symptoms, the better. Capsules are taken a piece or two at a time every four hours once an infection sets in before gradually tapering off the dose in the following days when symptoms improve.

Studies on goldenseal

Goldenseal contains berberine, a chemical that acts like a natural antimicrobial which can inhibit the growth of bacteria and fungi. It can also lower blood pressure and regulate erratic heartbeats aside from lowering blood sugar and bad cholesterol in the body's circulation. However, many of the potent chemicals of goldenseal are destroyed once they pass the digestive tract and it has yet to be proven that goldenseal actually has the same benefits as pure berberine. Some herbs such as the Chinese goldthread and Oregon grape have berberine and have been used as a substitute for its roots. There has yet to be any comprehensive study that can verify whether goldenseal is effective for any of its alleged benefits.

Other components found in goldenseal are hydrastine, the yellow coloring that makes up about two to four per cent of its alkaloid content, and canadine. The prized rhizomes are often rich in these alkaloids compared to what can be extracted from the roots.

References:

•   Discovery Health. "Discovery Health "Goldenseal: Herbal Remedies"." 2007. http://health.howstuffworks.com/wellness/natural-medicine/herbal-remedies/goldenseal-herbal-remedies.htm (accessed 10 Jun 2013).

•   Drugs.com. "Goldenseal Facts and Comparisons at Drugs.com." 2013. http://www.drugs.com/cdi/goldenseal.html (accessed 10 Jun 2013).

•   National Center for Complementary and Alternative Medicine (NCCAM). "Goldenseal | NCCAM." 2006. http://nccam.nih.gov/health/goldenseal (accessed 10 Jun 2013).

• University of Maryland Medical Center. "Goldenseal." 2012. http://www.umm.edu/altmed/articles/goldenseal-000252.htm (accessed 10 Jun 2013).

• WebMD. "GOLDENSEAL: Uses, Side Effects, Interactions and Warnings - WebMD." 2009. http://www.webmd.com/vitamins-supplements/ingredientmono-943-GOLDENSEAL.aspx?activeIngredientId=943&activeIngredientName=GOLDENSEAL (accessed 10 Jun 2013).

HAWTHORN- Hawthorn is a small tree whose berries, leaves, and flowers are used for herbal medication. The collective term describes the Crataegus oxycantha, Crataegus monogyna, and other similar species. It is also called aubepine, maythorn, quick thorn, white thorn, and haw. The genus name Crataegus comes from the Greek words "kratos" (which means hard, the quality of its wood), "oxcus" (meaning sharp), and akantha (denotes the thorns).

Growing hawthorn

There are as many as 280 species of hawthorn that exist but there are species that have been used for commercial manufacturing. This plant is related to the rose family. In general, hawthorn plants are thorny small trees that grow up to 7.5 metres high. The leaves are lobed and it has white fragrant flowers in bunches which bloom from April to June. Its bright, red fruit may contain nuts, depending on the species. The berries which sprout after the flowers are called haws. These are red or black when ripe.

Hawthorn has been used by Greek physicians for its diuretic effect, which is beneficial for kidney and bladder problems. In Europe, hawthorn supplements are utilised for blood pressure and heart rhythm. The leaves and flowers are approved in the Complete German Commission E Monographs as chronic treatment for heart failure type I and II. American physicians have used it for circulatory and respiratory conditions.

Benefits of hawthorn

Hawthorn has benefited circulatory conditions such as congestive heart failure, crushing chest pain, and erratic heartbeats. It has also been employed for extreme blood pressure, easing out the plaque in arteries, and keeping levels of bad cholesterol in check. Aside from these, the hawthorn extracts have also been utilised for digestive problems such as indigestion, loose bowel movements, and stomach upset. It has also been given as treatment for intestinal infestations such as those of tapeworms. Other benefits that can be derived from hawthorn are its calming effects for anxious patients, regulate menstruation, and act as diuretic for people suffering from oedema or hypertension. It has been given for skin conditions such as boils, sores, ulcers, itchy skin, and frostbite.

What to look out for

In general, hawthorn supplements are expected to be safe in adults when taken in label recommended doses for up to four months. There are no available data that show hawthorn is safe to use for a long time. No data is also available whether the plant extract is safe for breastfeeding and pregnant women. This supplement should never be given to children.

Common side effects associated with the use of hawthorn supplements are stomach upset, fatigue, headache, sweating, dizziness, palpitations, nosebleeds, and insomnia.

Hawthorn can interact with many medications that are used for treating heart disease. Antihypertensive medications such as atenolol, verapamil, amlodipine, and other similar drugs might drop blood pressure to dangerously low levels. Heart medications such as digoxin, nitroglycerin, and isosorbide might become more potent than usual with hawthorn, making side effects such as dizziness and fainting more pronounced. Drugs for erectile dysfunction (ED) such as sildenafil and the like might also cause blood pressure to drop dangerously low.

How to use hawthorn

Specific hawthorn supplements have been used for heart failure. Daily doses of 160 to 1800 milligrams are divided in two to three equal doses. These doses have been determined by studies sponsored by their manufacturers. According to studies, a minimum of 300 milligrams of standardised hawthorn extracts are given daily with its effects visible by two months of therapy. Fluid extracts of the berries may be given at 10 to 15 drops per dose. The combined tincture of flowers and herbs may be given at 2.5 millilitres to a teaspoon thrice a day.

Hawthorn is available in capsules and extracts in tincture and powdered forms. Other people prefer the dried or fresh berries which they can snack on. A bitter tea can be made from dried hawthorn leaves, flowers, and berries. A liqueur has been made from hawthorn berries with brandy. There are also online recipes on how to make hawthorn berry jam which can also do double duty as syrup. Tinctures from flowers are usually made in spring while those from berries are made during the fall. When mixed together, a potent mixture is made that can be combined with other heart tonic herbs such as garlic and motherwort.

Studies on hawthorn

Hawthorn leaves, flowers, bark, and berries are rich in flavonoids, proanthocyanidins, tyramine, and tannins. The first two are the most active medicinal substances found in hawthorn which have been standardised and used in scientific studies. About 2.2 per cent of flavonoids or 18.75 per cent oligomeric proanthocyanidines have been employed in trials. The berries contain amygdalin while the bark contains crataegin. Its brightly colored berries are rich in antioxidants, especially vitamin C.

There are some evidence that hawthorn can enhance the volume of blood pumped through the heart during its contractions, expand the blood vessels, and hasten nerve impulse transmission. Early studies have shown hawthorn's potential to control hypertension. Its proanthocyanidin content seems to lower blood pressure by relaxing blood vessels that are farthest from the heart. According to a separate study, hawthorn supplements are somewhat more effective than digoxin in managing congestive heart failure although the exact mechanism is unknown.

Research has also found a hint that hawthorn berries can lower bad cholesterol and freely circulating fats in the bloodstream. It does so by multiplying bile excretion which then lowers cholesterol manufacture and making receptors for bad cholesterol more sensitive to bind them and ship them out the body.

Hawthorn shows promise in stabilising collagen and in keeping cancer cells in check. There are triterpenes such as uvaol and ursolic acid that has been able to kill certain types of throat cancers in both humans and rats. The exact mechanism is still unknown.

There are some data that has shown hawthorn extracts, when combined with magnesium and California poppy, have been somewhat remedial for mild to moderate anxiety. Animal studies have shown hawthorn's potential as an herbal analgesic and anxiolytic.

References:

• A Modern Herbal. "A Modern Herbal | Hawthorn." n.d.. http://botanical.com/botanical/mgmh/h/hawtho09.html (accessed 10 Jun 2013).

• Drugs.com. "Hawthorn professional information from Drugs.com." 2010. http://www.drugs.com/npp/hawthorn.html (accessed 10 Jun 2013).

- National Center for Complementary and Alternative Medicine (NCCAM). "Hawthorn | NCCAM." 2006. http://nccam.nih.gov/health/hawthorn (accessed 10 Jun 2013).

- WebMD. "Hawthorn: Uses, Side Effects, Interactions and Warnings - WebMD." 2009. http://www.webmd.com/vitamins-supplements/ingredientmono-527-hawthorn.aspx?activeIngredientId=527&activeIngredientName=hawthorn (accessed 10 Jun 2013).

- University of Maryland Medical Center. "Hawthorn." 2012. http://www.umm.edu/altmed/articles/hawthorn-000256.htm (accessed 10 Jun 2013).

HOP - Hop is a climbing, flowering vine that is related to hemp and hackberries. Its scientific name is Humulus lupulus and is also known for its common names asperge sauvage, hopfenzapfen, houblon, pi jiu hua, and hops. The plant is a popular ingredient for beers and other beverages, especially in the Middle Ages. This herb is a native of Great Britain.

Growing hop

Hops have been used for many years as a flavouring and preservative for beer, especially at a time when drinking beer is safer than untreated water. This herb is a native of the Northern Hemispheres and will grow exuberantly from April to July in temperate climates. Wild hop can be found in shrubs and forest edge with adequate supply of water and require deep, fertile soil with good drainage. Cultivated hops bear their goods after their third year.

Since the hop flowers only bloom at certain latitudes, there are limited regions where it can be cultivated. Flowers are cultivated and are often prevented from having their fruits from ripening. It is often harvested from August to September in the North while it's scheduled in February for those grown in the South.

Benefits of hop

Aside from being a major ingredient of liquors and beers, hop is employed for its calming and relaxing effect. It has also benefited people with poor appetites or digestion, increases urine excretion, and helps improve breast milk flow. It has been employed for certain cancers, control of bad cholesterol levels, and cramps in the intestines. Its antimicrobial properties have been useful for people with tuberculosis, colitis, and leg ulcers. Since it can relieve aches, it has also been used for nerve pain and persistent, painful penile erection.

What to look out for

In general, hop is likely safe for most people. However, there is no present data that proves hops are safe for pregnant and breastfeeding women. Taking supplements that contain hop might worsen cases of depression. People who are scheduled for surgery should stop taking the herb a fortnight before your appointment on the operating table. Hops might worsen drowsiness once anaesthesia and other medications are infused in the circulation.

Aside from its sedative effect, hop extracts might also trigger rash and breathing difficulty, as observed from its harvesters. People with allergy to peanuts, chestnuts, and bananas should keep away from using this herb. Consuming too much hop will cause seizures, fevers, restlessness, vomiting, and hyperacidity. Ironically, hop extracts can lower blood sugar of normal people but will spike blood sugar in those suffering from diabetes.

Alcohol and hops might make one very sleepy more than when taking any of them alone. It might also cause the same effect with sedatives and antidepressants such as lorazepam, barbiturates, zolpidem, and other similar medications. Medications that affect hormones such as those for diabetes, oral contraceptives, or hormone replacement therapy might interact with this supplement. People taking cholesterol-lowering supplements such as guggul and red yeast might experience additive effects with hop that has a similar action.

How to use hop

There is a supplement that combines 41.9 milligrams of hop with 187 milligrams of valerian per tablet. This is given for people with difficulty sleeping. Two tablets are taken at bedtime and it will take about less than a month to ease up on sleep. Two weeks treatment of such supplement does not seem to improve sleeping pattern. Another similar combination involves hops in combination with its dried strobile, where doses of 1.5 to two grams are given before bedtime.

An infusion of hop may have sedative properties but it has been used in folk medicine as a tonic for heart conditions, nervous disorders, and afflictions of the digestive system. Its bitter principles are good digestive tonics. It has also been used to calm an irritated bladder. When this infusion is mixed with chamomile flowers or poppy heads, it can act as an analgesic for anything swollen and sore. It can also be applied as a poultice for bruises, boils, and swollen joints. A warmed pillow made of hops is believed to ease pains of the ear and the tooth while exerting a calming effect.

Studies on hop

There are chemicals in hops that exhibit slight oestrogenic effects. It has bitter principles such as colupulone and humulone, the latter which gives beer its characteristic bitter taste. Hops also contain essential oils which may contain mostly caryophyllene, myrcene, and humulene. It also contains flavonoids such as xanthohumol and prenylnaringenin, the latter being attributed for hop's alleged oestrogen-like abilities.

Hop pickers have often experienced drowsiness during harvest which spurred a series of research on hop's sedative abilities. Animal studies have been promising but when tested on humans, valerian is more potent and far more effective as a sleep aid than hop.

Scientists have long suspected hop to be a plant with oestrogen-like abilities. This was further proven with 100 micrograms prenylnaringenin dissolved in 100 millilitres of drinking water was able to affect animal uteri. It was also observed during hop's evaluation in treating menstrual symptoms. This was exploited by supplements claiming it can enhance women's breasts when it can trigger liver and pancreatic hormonal problems in rats.

The bitter acids in hop have shown significant effects on metabolic enzymes. Colupulone and humulone have been tested on its abilities to stop tumour production using assays and animal studies. Humulone and its derivatives, especially xanthohumol, have shown potential in stopping tumour development and spread in animals. In spite of this, there are no clinical data that has shown hop can prevent cancer.

Traditionally, the addition of hop extracts in beer for flavour and preservation have been attributed to the herb's antimicrobial ability. Isohumolone has demonstrated its ability to limit the bacterial population in beer. Its prenylflavonoids have shown to be better antioxidants than any other components in hop. Humulone is being studied as a possible cyclooxygenase-2 (COX-2) inhibitor. Although hop has been used for a variety of conditions, there has yet to be a large scale investigation on its benefits.

References:

- American Botanical Council. "HerbalGram: Hops (Humulus lupulus): A Review of its Historic and Medicinal Uses." 2009. http://cms.herbalgram.org/herbalgram/issue87/article3559.html (accessed 11 Jun 2013).

- Drugs.com. "Hops professional information from Drugs.com." 2001. http://www.drugs.com/npp/hops.html (accessed 11 Jun 2013).

- Healthline. "What is Hops? Dosing, Side Effects & More." 2004. http://www.healthline.com/natstandardcontent/hops (accessed 11 Jun 2013).

- Plant Profiler. "Hops (Humulus lupulus) | Plant Profiler." 2010. http://www.sigmaaldrich.com/life-science/nutrition-research/learning-center/plant-profiler/humulus-lupulus.html (accessed 11 Jun 2013).

- WebMD. "HOPS: Uses, Side Effects, Interactions and Warnings - WebMD." 2009. http://www.webmd.com/vitamins-supplements/ingredientmono-856-HOPS.aspx?activeIngredientId=856&activeIngredientName=HOPS (accessed 11 Jun 2013).

HORSE CHESTNUT- Horse chestnut is a large tree whose bark, leaves, and fruit have been used as herbal medicine. Its scientific name is Aesculus hippocastanum and is sometimes referred to by other common names such as aescin, conker tree, white chestnut, and buckeye. This tree has often been confused with other related species such as the California and the Ohio buckeye.

Growing horse chestnut

Horse chestnuts are native trees that are abundant in Greece, Bulgaria, and north central parts of Asia but have spread throughout the Northern Hemisphere. The name horse chestnut comes from its appearance that looks like the edible, sweet chestnuts but are "gwres," which means pungent and bitter, for the inedible nuts. Its branches have marks that are similar to minute horseshoes.

The tree trunks of the horse chestnut are straight and tall, with wide spreading branches. Its smooth, greyish green bark has been used as yellow dye and hides the soft and spongy wood. Its large leaves are spread like fingers and have finely toothed margins. Its white flowers have a reddish mark. The fruit of the tree is a shiny, brown nut, with large green husk and covered with short spines that split when the nut falls to the ground.

The horse chestnut can be cultivated from its nuts that have been gathered in autumn. These are sown in early spring and will grow with little care on sandy loam soil.

Benefits of horse chestnut

Extracts from the horse chestnut seeds and leaves are often indicated for those suffering from varicose veins, haemorrhoids, and engorged veins. Horse chestnut seeds have been employed for diarrhoea, fever, and distended prostate. When its active principles are extracted and concentrated, the horse chestnut seed can be utilised for chronic venous insufficiency. The leaves of the horse chestnut have been given for eczema, menstrual pain, swelling from bone fractures and sprains, and arthritis. Its bark has been applied on the skin for lupus and ulcers or infused to relieve symptoms of malaria and dysentery. It also has narcotic and a febrifuge when consumed orally.

What to look out for

When standard seed extracts are taken according to labelled instructions and used short term the seeds of the horse chestnut are relatively safe. Use only products that have verified standardised horse chestnut components and stay away from those that have not removed esculin, a toxic substance in the seeds, from the supplements. Sometimes, people who take horse chestnut will experience headaches, itching, stomach discomfort, and being lightheaded. Rectal formulations containing horse chestnut extracts might cause swelling and itching of the anus.

Fresh horse chestnut flowers have pollen that might cause hypersensitivity in certain individuals. Raw horse chestnut seeds, bark, flowers, and leaves are poisonous and lethally toxic when taken by mouth. Children have been poisoned just by drinking tea made from fresh leaves and twig or have accidentally eaten its seeds.

Since there are no data that shows processed horse chestnut extracts are safe for pregnant and breastfeeding women, it's best to stay out of harm's way and not use the product. It might contain trace amounts of esculin which could be harmful for the foetus or nursing infant. There are some conditions that should be careful when using horse chestnut supplements. Diabetics should monitor their blood sugar regularly as this plant can lower blood sugar to dangerously low levels. People suffering from liver, digestive tract, and kidney diseases might have their condition worsen.

Horse chestnut extracts might also interact with other medications. Since it has a slight diuretic effect, the side effects of lithium might be more pronounced than usual. Its ability to lower blood sugar can also potentiate the effect of anti-diabetic drugs such as glimepride, insulin, rosiglitazone, glipizide, and other similar drugs. The seeds of the horse chestnut are natural blood thinners so using anticoagulant and antiplatelet drugs and some non-steroidal anti-inflammatory drugs as aspirin, naproxen, and the like might increase the risk for bruising and uncontrolled bleeding.

How to use horse chestnut

Most of the doses used for horse chestnut are determined by the labelled instruction by the supplement manufacturers and should be followed carefully. However, there are doses based on the ones used in scientific research where horse chestnut supplements are found to be effective.

Doses of 50 milligrams aescin, an active ingredient found in the seeds, are given every 12 hours to improve blood circulation in people suffering from chronic venous insufficiency. Alternatively, a dose of 250 to 750 milligrams per day may be given in divided doses. It should never be chewed and taken with a full glass of water. Tinctures are often given at one to four millilitres every eight hours. A tincture of the bark may be given in an infusion of an ounce of bark to a pint of water. A tablespoonful is every three to four times a day or applied topically to ulcers.

There are some topical applications containing horse chestnut that are used to improve the appearance of unsightly varicose veins and applied on swollen joints, muscles, and haemorrhoids. The cream or gel should be applied on clean, dried affected area before applying the topical preparation thinly. It should never be applied on broken skin and mucous membranes.

Studies on horse chestnut

Horse chestnut contains saponins, the most important of these is aescin, which acts like a vasoconstrictor. It also has aesculin, a type of hydroxycoumarin that thins out blood by limiting thrombin.

The active constituents of the horse chestnut have prevented fluids from leaking out of blood vessels. There are studies that have provided evidence that poor blood circulation can be improved by horse chestnut extracts. Varicose veins, throbbing pain, and swollen legs are some of the symptoms that seem to respond well with the plant. Its effectiveness has been compared to the benefits gained from wearing compression stockings.

There is insufficient evidence that horse chestnut is effective for haemorrhoids, diarrhoea, fever, cough, distended prostate, eczema, menstrual pain, and swelling from bone fractures and sprains, including those caused by arthritis.

References:

- A Modern Herbal. "Chestnut, Horse." 2013. http://botanical.com/botanical/mgmh/c/chehor58.html (accessed 11 Jun 2013).

- Drugs.com. "Horse chestnut medical facts from Drugs.com." 2010. http://www.drugs.com/mtm/horse-chestnut.html (accessed 11 Jun 2013).

- Medline Plus. "Horse chestnut: MedlinePlus Supplements." 2004. http://www.nlm.nih.gov/medlineplus/druginfo/natural/1055.html (accessed 11 Jun 2013).

- Medscape. "Medscape: Medscape Access." 2013. http://reference.medscape.com/drug/aescin-aesculaforce-horse-chestnut-seed-344492 (accessed 11 Jun 2013).

- National Center for Complementary and Alternative Medicine (NCCAM). "Horse Chestnut | NCCAM." 2006. http://nccam.nih.gov/health/horsechestnut (accessed 11 Jun 2013).

HYSSOP – Hyssop is a large shrub that has a scientific name of Hyssopus officinalis. It is also known for its common names herbe de Joseph, herbe sainte, hiope, hisopo, jufa, and rabo de gato. It is a local plant of southern Europe, Middle East, and countries surrounding the Caspian Sea. It has been mentioned a lot of time in the Christian bible as a sacred herb.

Growing hyssop

Hyssop is a brilliantly colorful shrub that can grow to about two feet in height. The stem is often woody at the base with slender, green leaves that are about an inch long. Its stems are somewhat hairy and have purple blue flowers. In the summer, this plant will bloom colorful and fragrant flowers which eventually form small, grape-like fruit. It is resistant to drought and can survive on dusty, sandy soil. It grows well in full sunlight and warm climates.

The plant can be grown from its seeds, usually in April, or through cuttings which are planted in spring under a shady area. When planted in a warm area with light, somewhat dry soil, the plant needs consistent watering until fully grown. The flowers bloom from June to October.

When the weather is good, hyssop can be harvested twice a year, usually at the end of spring and at the beginning of fall. The herb is picked while it is flowering to collect the flowering tips, usually in August. The stalks are then cut and dried in cool, dry, ventilated areas, away from the sun, for about a week. Once dried, the leaves are trimmed and chopped finely before being stored where it can keep for 18 months. Its oil is extracted from leaves and flower buds through steam distillation.

Benefits of hyssop

Hyssop has been given for problems of the digestive system such as liver and gallbladder disorders, gas, colic, stomach pain, and poor appetite. It has also been prescribed for infections of the urinary tract (UTI) and human immunodeficiency virus (HIV), poor blood circulation, and menstrual cramps. It has been prescribed for its ability to release excess gas and cramping in the stomach, remove excess phlegm, work up a sweat, calm the nerves, diminish swollen and sore muscles and joints, and stimulate menstruation.

Its astringent effect keeps the skin from sagging and helps teeth stay in place. It also helps heal deep cuts and improve the appearance of scars, especially those caused by boils, pox, insect bites, and infections. The hyssop extracts can also raise blood pressure and tones up the nervous system. It can also eliminate some worms from the body. The oil can be used in aromatherapy.

What to look out for

If taken in amounts used for food or in dosages indicated in the supplement's label, hyssop is generally safe. The oil formulation should not be used because it might cause seizures in some people sensitive to its components. Children should steer clear of hyssop as there are cases where two to three drops taken for several days cause convulsions. People who have a history of seizures should never use hyssop as it might trigger an attack or make it worse than usual.

How to use hyssop

Fresh hyssop is used in cooking as an aromatic condiment. Its leaves have a light bitter taste with a minty smell. The intense flavour has had its use to a minimal in cooking. Sometimes, the oils are also used for cooking.

Traditionally, hyssop is used to cough out phlegm and expel gas in the intestine. Fresh tops of the leaves are boiled in soup and given to people who suffer from asthma. Alternatively, it can be given as a warm infusion or mixed with another herb, horehound or coltsfoot for coughs and bronchitis. On the other hand, the infusion of hyssop leaves is given to relieve rheumatism, bruises, and contusion. Freshly bruised or crumbled leaves applied on wounds and cuts are believed to heal immediately. A fluid extract of hyssop is given at 1.5 to three millilitres per dose.

Studies on hyssop

Hyssop contains terpinoids such as marrubin, oleanolic and ursolic acids. It also has volatile oils that are a mix of camphor, pinocaphone, thujone, isopinocamphone, linalool, bornyl acetate, and terpinenene among many others. It is also rich in flavonoids such as diosmin and hesperidin. Other identified active ingredients are hyssopin, a glucoside, some tannin, and a resin.

Hyssop contains chemicals that can affect the heart and stimulate the lungs to produce more secretions. The plant is a member of the mint family and is abundant in chemicals found in related plants. Its fragrant, volatile chemicals are made up of camphone, pinene, camphene, and terpinene which make up about 70 per cent of the volatile oil. Other components of hyssop are glycosides such as hyssopin, hesperidin, and diosmin, tannins, oleanolic and ursolic acids, sitosterol, marrubin, and resins. In addition, other identified compounds are pinocampheol, cineole, linalool, terpineol, pinic, pinonic, and myrtenic acids, and cadinene. Crude extracts of hyssop have been found to contain rosmarinic acid and hydroxycinnamic derivatives.

It has been determined that the apparent neurotoxicity of hyssop extracts is caused by the terpene ketones pinocamphone and isopinocamphone. This was proven in a rat experiment where the essential oils are enough to trigger convulsions that can lead to death. Its oleanolic and ursolic acids have been studied for its ability to lower lipids in circulation. The diosmin and hesperidin content have been found in clinical trials to improve chronic venous insufficiency and control blood sugar in Type I diabetics. Its marrubin content has shown promise in some studies as an alternative expectorant and increases secretion of bile, but in test animals.

There is insufficient evidence that hyssop and its extracts are effective for conditions such as colds, sore throat or asthma. It also lacks data for hyssop's usefulness in liver, gallbladder, and intestinal problems aside from colic and poor appetite. There has yet to be enough studies that can prove hyssop can claim to be effective against UTI and HIV.

References:

• Botanical.com. "A Modern Herbal | Hyssop." 2013. http://botanical.com/botanical/mgmh/h/hyssop48.html (accessed 12 Jun 2013).

• Drugs.com. "Hyssop professional information from Drugs.com." 2002. http://www.drugs.com/npp/hyssop.html (accessed 12 Jun 2013).

• Plant Profiler. "Hyssop (Hyssopus officinalis) | Plant Profiler." 2010. http://www.sigmaaldrich.com/life-science/nutrition-research/learning-center/plant-profiler/hyssopus-officinalis.html (accessed 12 Jun 2013).

• RxList. "Hyssop Effectiveness, Safety, and Drug Interactions on RxList." 2013. http://www.rxlist.com/hyssop/supplements.htm (accessed 12 Jun 2013).

@Arthur Bramble@

WebMD. "HYSSOP: Uses, Side Effects, Interactions and Warnings - WebMD." 2009. http://www.webmd.com/vitamins-supplements/ingredientmono-258-HYSSOP.aspx?activeIngredientId=258&activeIngredientName=HYSSOP (accessed 12 Jun 2013).

HERBAL REMEDIES I-P

JUNIPER- Juniper is a type of evergreen tree with blue or reddish berry-like cones are used as herbal medicine. Its scientific name is Juniperus communis and is also known as enebro, genievre, wacholderbeeren, and zimbro. The Navajo Indians have used the berries for diabetes while other tribes use it as a contraceptive for females.

Growing juniper

Juniper trees are native to Northern Europe, Asia, and North America. It is a small tree which can grow up to four to six feet in height. It grows under full sun on chalky slopes or on fertile, little traces of lime, silicon rich soil. These are coniferous trees that bear cones; only in this case, their cones look more like berries as it has fleshier scales.

Juniper berries might take about two to three years to ripen. Only the blue ones are harvested and used, leaving the green ones to ripen. The parts often used are its ripe, dried fruits and leaves. Commercial grade juniper oil comes from the ripe berries while those valued for its medicinal properties come from the unripe ones. The latter produces a pale, greenish-yellow, clear liquid that is somewhat turpentine-like odour when fresh, and has an oily, resinous, stinging, and slightly bitter taste.

Benefits of juniper

Juniper has been a traditional flavouring ingredient in foods and in alcoholic liquors such as gin. The juniper extracts are mixed in with the gin as a remedy for kidney problems. The berries have also been used as seasoning for pickled meat or in sauces and stuffings. It has been employed in perfumes and cosmetics. It has been used in aromatherapy for its cleansing, calming effect. Some cultures have used it as healing incense, such as the Native Americans.

The juniper extracts have been employed for its ability to release gas, bloating, heartburn, bloating and poor appetite. Some people have utilised its oils as a steam inhalant to manage bronchitis. Swiss medicine has employed this plant to treat wounds and inflamed conditions, such as arthritis, for its analgesic effect. The irritating effect it exerts on the bladder has made it an effective diuretic for those suffering from urinary tract infection (UTI) and kidney stones but has been limited to low concentrations. It has also been given for snakebites and intestinal worms.

What to look out for

When used for a short period of time, juniper is generally safe for most adults. Use it longer than a month and it might damage the kidneys and seizures. When applied on small areas of the skin or inhaling its vapours, juniper is somewhat safe as some allergies on the skin and the respiratory system might happen when using juniper berries or any of its extracts. It might cause irritation, stinging, redness, and swelling.

Juniper extracts have also caused a dip in the blood sugar levels of experimental animals. It is a major concern that it might also cause the same effect on diabetic humans. It can also cause extremes in blood pressure which can make hypertension a little difficult to manage. Because of such effects, stop using juniper extracts a fortnight before any scheduled surgery or dental procedure.

There are available data that documents juniper's ability to cause extreme catharsis, urination, and spasms of the uterus in large doses of the extract. Breastfeeding and pregnant women should never use this herbal supplement. People with problems in their kidneys should also avoid using anything with juniper extracts.

Juniper can affect medications that are used for managing diabetes. It can potentiate the hypoglycemic effect of glyburide, insulin, rosiglitazone, glipizide, and other similar medications. Monitor blood sugar levels regularly. It can also dehydrate the body when used in conjunction with water pills such as chorothiazide, furosemide, hydrodiuril, and other similar medications.

How to use juniper

There are no standard doses for juniper extracts. Traditionally, a 0.1 millilitre or about 20 to 100 milligrams of the essential oil is given for dyspepsia. About 2 or 10 grams of the berry is taken for juniper's use as a diuretic or to stimulate menstruation.

Those taking juniper extracts in capsules should follow the manufacturer's labelled instructions, usually given at 800 milligrams every 12 hours. People who prefer consuming juniper berries will find it effective at one or two grams thrice a day. A teaspoon of about two to three grams of the crushed berry steeped in 150 millilitres of boiling water will make a cup of juniper tea that can be taken thrice daily. A liquid extract of juniper berries dissolved in one part of 25 per cent alcohol or a tincture of juniper dissolved in five parts of 45 per cent alcohol may be taken at two to four millilitres every eight hours

Studies on juniper

The essential oil of the juniper berries are made up mostly of monoterpenes such as pinene, sabinene, limonene, terpineol, borneol, geraniol, myrcene, camphene, camphor, and eudesmol. It also has sesquiterpenes that are made up of caryophyllene, cadinene, muurolene, humulene, and pregeijerene. Aside from these, it also contains diterpenes such as sugiol, xanthoperol, and abietic, palustric, communic, and sandracopimaric acid. It is also rich in flavonoids such as isocutellarein, hypolaetin, kaempferol, quercitin, nicotiflorin, and naringenin. The lignan podophyllotoxin has been identified to be poisonous to the nerves, gut, and liver. Its eudesmol content has shown to hinder the usual mechanism of calcium channels and in doing so, becomes neuroprotective in stroke patients. Odiolactone has been identified as its antifungal compound while the isocrupressic acid is an active abortifacient. The tannin content has an astringent effect.

According to some studies, juniper berries have chemicals that can lower inflammation and release excess gas. It has been studied for its effectiveness to keep bacterial and viral infections at bay. There is also some proof that it has a diuretic effect. However, there is not enough evidence that shows it can actually be effective for upset stomach, heartburn, bloating, poor appetite, UTIs, kidney stones, joint and muscle pain, and wounds. Its diuretic effect has been attributed to its terpinene-4-ol compound.

References:

• A Modern Herbal. "A Modern Herbal | Juniper Berries." 2005. http://botanical.com/botanical/mgmh/j/junipe11.html (accessed 12 Jun 2013).

• Drugs.com. "Juniper information from Drugs.com." 2004. http://www.drugs.com/npc/juniper.html (accessed 12 Jun 2013).

• Medscape. "Medscape: Medscape Access." 2013. http://reference.medscape.com/drug/juniperus-communis-juniper-344563 (accessed 12 Jun 2013).

• RxList. "Juniper Effectiveness, Safety, and Drug Interactions on RxList." 2013. http://www.rxlist.com/juniper/supplements.htm (accessed 12 Jun 2013).

WebMD. "JUNIPER: Uses, Side Effects, Interactions and Warnings - WebMD." 2009. http://www.webmd.com/vitamins-supplements/ingredientmono-724-JUNIPER.aspx?activeIngredientId=724&activeIngredientName=JUNIPER (accessed 12 Jun 2013).

LAVENDER- Lavender is a shrub whose flowers and oils are used as plant remedy. It's a collective term for a variety of fragrant flowering species related to the mint. However, the Lavandula angustifolia or the common lavender is the most commonly used species for herbal medications. It has also been known as Lavandula officinalis or Lavandula vera. It has been called as alhucema and ostokhoddous in other languages. The name comes from the Latin word "lavare," which means to wash as the herb has been used in baths.

Growing lavender

The common lavender is a native plant of the western Mediterranean. It can grow up to about three to six feet tall and produce pinkish purple flowers that are found as spikes on the very top of the willowy, leaf bare stems. The term angustifolia refers to its very narrow leaves.

The lavender has been cultivated mainly for its ornamental purpose. It has beautiful, fragrant flowers that can thrive even on poorly watered soil. It can tolerate low temperatures and acidic soil. It has been used in ancient Egypt for its mummification process while it is a bath additive in Persia, Greece, and Rome.

Benefits of lavender

Lavender is a soothing, calming herb for anxiety, sleeplessness, tensions, and depression. It has been prescribed for digestive complaints such as bloating, poor appetite, vomiting and nausea, flatulence, and stomach upset. The extracts have been given for pain and swelling such as migraine headaches, toothaches, sprains, joint pain, and even swabbed on wounds and sores. It also benefits the skin as it may treat acne, hair loss, and as insect repellent. Some people add lavender on their bathwater to improve circulation and mental well-being or inhaled in aromatherapy for insomnia, anxiety, pain, and restlessness caused by dementia.

What to look out for

In general, lavender is generally safe for most adults when taken in the usual amounts for food or in the labelled amount for herbal supplements. When taken orally, lavender might cause constipation, headache, and an increase in appetite. If applied directly on skin, lavender might cause irritation.

Products that contain lavender might not be safe for male children who have not reached puberty. The herb has a hormone-like effect on the male hormones which might cause abnormal breast growth known as gynecomastia. The effects of this product on female children have not been studied. Oral use is not recommended for children. Pregnant and breastfeeding women should stay away from the use of lavender as there are no studies showing the safety of its use.

Lavender might slow down nerve impulses of the central nervous system (CNS). When used in combination with anaesthesia used in surgery, it might slow down the CNS and deteriorate into a comatose state. If you can, stop lavender use at least two weeks before the scheduled surgery or dental procedure.

Lavender supplements might interact with medications that have a sedative effect. It might lead to excessive sleepiness and drowsiness that might affect concentration and focus. Some medications to watch out for are phenobarbital, lorazepam, zolpidem, and other similar medications.

How to use lavender

The flowers and leaves are the parts of the lavender are used as herbal medication. They are expressed for their oil or used as herbal tea. Lavender oil can be mixed with carrier oils and used for massage and aromatherapy. The flowers can be used in cooking and a major ingredient of a French herbal mix known as herbes de Provence. The flower stalks have been used for deodorising the air.

For bald spots, a mixture of lavender, rosemary, thyme, and cedarwood in jojoba and grapeseed oil as base is massaged on the balding part of the scalp for two minutes and a warm towel placed around the head for better absorption. Add two to four drops of lavender oil in two to three cups of boiling water. The vapours may be inhaled for relief of headache, insomnia, or depression. About one to four drops of lavender dissolved per tablespoon of almond or olive oil may be applied on the skin.

Studies on lavender

The volatile oil of the lavender gives it medicinal properties. The dried flowers will yield pale yellow to colorless oil with fragrance similar to flowers and a slightly bitter taste. It contains seven to ten per cent linalool and linanlyl acetate, which is also found in bergamot oil. Other substances identified in the oil are cineol, pinene, limonene, geraniol, and borneol with trace amounts of tannins.

There is some evidence that lavender oil actually has a sedating effect which can provide specific muscle relaxation. However, the tincture of lavender was not able to improve mild to moderate depression compared to imipramine. There are some data that demonstrated rubbing two to three drops of lavender oil on the upper lip was able to lower the intensity of migraine pain, nausea, and prevent the headache from spreading.

Lavender is possibly effective for a hair loss condition known as alopecia areata. When combined with other oils such as thyme, rosemary, and cedarwood, lavender oil can improve hair growth by about 44 per cent after seven months of use. There is initial research is being developed that suggests that inhaling lavender oil, whether through a bedside diffuser or gauze, overnight might help people affected with mild insomnia.

There are contradictory data whether lavender is beneficial for anxiety in people suffering from dementia. There is a study where nightly use of lavender diffuser for three weeks has been able to reduce the incidence of agitation. In a separate study, the continuous of lavender steeped pad attached on the subject's shirt were not able to lower the incidence of excitement in those with advanced dementia. There is a study that demonstrated a mix of 20 per cent lavender to 80 per cent grapeseed oil added to daily baths were able to improve positive well-being compared to grapeseed alone.

More evidence is needed to prove lavender is effective for colic, poor appetite, acne, cancer, and as insect repellent.

References:

- A Modern Herbal. "A Modern Herbal | Lavenders." 2004. http://botanical.com/botanical/mgmh/l/lavend13.html (accessed 13 Jun 2013).

- Medline Plus. "Lavender: MedlinePlus Supplements." 2012. http://www.nlm.nih.gov/medlineplus/druginfo/natural/83 8.html (accessed 13 Jun 2013).

- National Center for Complementary and Alternative Medicine (NCCAM). "Lavender | NCCAM." 2007. http://nccam.nih.gov/health/lavender/ataglance.htm (accessed 13 Jun 2013).

- University of Maryland Medical Center. "Lavender." 2007. http://umm.edu/health/medical/altmed/herb/lavender (accessed 13 Jun 2013).

- WebMD. "lavender: Uses, Side Effects, Interactions and Warnings - WebMD." 2009. http://www.webmd.com/vitamins-supplements/ingredientmono-838-lavender.aspx?activeIngredientId=838&activeIngredientNa me=lavender (accessed 13 Jun 2013).

LEMON BALM- Lemon balm is an herb that is related to the mint family. It is known for its scientific name Melissa officinalis and has been called by its common name balm mint, dropsy plant, honey plant, sweet balm, or sweet Mary. The name comes from the leaves which emit a subtle lemony fragrance. The small, white, nectar-rich flowers attract many bees, and the Greek term for bee is Melissa.

Growing lemon balm

The lemon balm is a native plant of south central Europe and the Mediterranean. In Northern America, the lemon balm has not been cultivated and grows mostly in the wild.

This herb can grow from two to four feet high. It needs some light and a 20 degree Centigrade temperature to grow. It often does so in clumps and will spread fast. In mildly temperate climates, the stems of the lemon balm dies out in winter and grow back in spring.

Benefits of lemon balm

Lemon balm is often given for digestive troubles such as stomach upset, bloating, gas, vomiting, and colic. It has also been employed for management of mild to moderate pain such as menstrual cramps, headache, and toothache. Its soothing effects is believed to benefit mental conditions such as hysteria, melancholia, anxiety, insomnia, restiveness, Alzheimer's disease, and attention deficit-hyperactivity disorder (ADHD). Some people affected with Grave's disease, sores, tumours, and insect bites benefit from using lemon balm extracts. It has also been applied to cold sores.

What to look out for

When taken as food, lemon balm is safe. If taken as an herbal medication, lemon balm is probably safe in adults when taken in small amounts. Infants have used it safely for a week while children under the age of 12 have been able to use it for a month. Researchers have used it for as long as four months without any harmful effects on the test subjects. Nevertheless, there is not enough data on lemon balm's safety when taken long term. To be on the safe side, breastfeeding and pregnant women should stay away from lemon balm use.

Lemon balm consumed might also cause some side effects such as queasiness, vomiting, abdominal pain, light-headedness, and breathlessness. When applied on the skin, there is a case of irritation and another report of recurrent cold sore symptoms. It should not be given to people with underactive thyroid.

Extracts of lemon balm can cause extreme drowsiness. It will interact with medications that are used for surgery and will cause extreme sleepiness. Stop using lemon balm two weeks before any scheduled surgery or dental procedure. Sedative medications such as clonazepam, phenobarbital, zolpidem and other similar medications may also become more potent when used with lemon balm.

How to use lemon balm

Some doses have been found effective in managing specific conditions. Traditionally, two to five grams of the leaves are steeped in 150 millilitres boiling water to make a cup of lemon balm tea taken when needed. It has also been steeped in wine to improve mood, heal wounds, and heal insect bites.

A dose of three millilitres of one part standardised lemon balm extract to one part 45 per cent alcohol is given for those with mild to moderate Alzheimer's disease. For those who want to sleep better, a combination of 80 milligrams lemon balm leaf extract and 160 milligrams valerian root extract, is given thrice daily for up to a month. Alternatively, the same formulation is also given for children, but once or twice daily.

For cases of mild to moderate dyspepsia, a combination of lemon balm and other herbs such as peppermint leaves, German chamomile, caraway, liquorice, clown mustard, celandine, angelica, and milk thistle, have been given for one millilitre every eight hours for a month. For colicky breastfed infants, a dose of 97 milligrams of lemon balm combined with 164 milligrams of fennel and 178 milligrams of German chamomile are given twice daily for 7 days.

A cream or ointment containing one per cent of lyophilised water soluble lemon balm extract is applied every six to 12 hours on cold sores. It may be given at the onset up a few days to a fortnight after it has healed.

Studies on lemon balm

Citronellal, geranial, linalyl acetate, and caryophyllene make up the lemon balm's distinct flavour. There are components that are said to have calming, sedative effects. It also has a mild, antiviral property.

Lemon balm's calming effects have been backed up by some studies. A study on lemon balm's effect on Alzheimer patients has been positive. A standardised extract of lemon balm given orally every day for four months was able to lessen the anxiety and other symptoms of Alzheimer's disease. There are also data that demonstrated that lemon balm extract mixed with valerian can greatly improve sleep quality. Another study on lemon balm involved its effect on colicky breastfed infants. The clinical trial used a mix of fennel, lemon balm, and German chamomile every 12 hours for a week and was able to shorten the babies' cries compared to other colicky babies. There is another research on the effects of lemon balm on people who suffer from dyspepsia. In this study, lemon balm is combined with peppermint, German chamomile, caraway, liquorice, clown's mustard, celandine, angelica, and milk thistle. This formulation has been able to relieve acid reflux, stomach aches and cramping, nausea, and vomiting. Lemon balm is also effective even when locally applied to cold sores. A one per cent concentration of lemon balm extract in lip balm was able to cut healing time in half, stop the spread of infection, and have milder recurrent cold sore symptoms.

Early data has implied that a tablet or two given once or twice daily of 80 milligram lemon balm leaf extract and 160 milligram valerian root extract was able to lower the excitability of children under 12 years of age. Despite of the possibilities lemon balm has in store, it needs more evidence on its claims that it can manage restlessness in children with ADHD.

References:

• A Modern Herbal. "A Modern Herbal | Balm." 1900. http://botanical.com/botanical/mgmh/b/balm--02.html (accessed 13 Jun 2013).

• Drugs.com. "Lemon Balm professional information from Drugs.com." 2008. http://www.drugs.com/npp/lemon-balm.html (accessed 13 Jun 2013).

• Medscape. "Lemon balm." 2013. http://reference.medscape.com/drug/balm-bee-balm-lemon-balm-344501 (accessed 13 Jun 2013).

• University of Maryland Medical Center. "Lemon balm." 2007. http://umm.edu/health/medical/altmed/herb/lemon-balm (accessed 13 Jun 2013).

WebMD. "LEMON BALM: Uses, Side Effects, Interactions and Warnings - WebMD." 2009. http://www.webmd.com/vitamins-supplements/ingredientmono-437-LEMON%20BALM.aspx?activeIngredientId=437&activeIngredientName=LEMON%20BALM (accessed 13 Jun 2013).

LICORICE- Licorice is a root of the legume Glycyrrhiza glabra. The name may be spelled as liquorice. It is also known by other names such as jethi-madh, kanzo, lakritze, mulathi, orozuz, reglisse, and sussholz. The name licorice comes from the Greek word glukurrhiza which means sweet root. It has been used by both traditional Eastern and Western medicine to heal common illnesses, although some of it might not have any scientific basis.

Growing licorice

Licorice is a native of Southern Europe and some parts of Asia. It can grow up to three to seven feet high but its roots can branch out extensively underground. Each root appear as long, cylindrical, wrinkled, fibrous wood that appear brown on the outside but yellowish on the inside. It has small purplish flowers that have pods often growing from its leaflets. The roots of the licorice are often harvested in the autumn of their fourth year. The roots and rhizomes are often exposed before being pulled out of the ground. It is then washed, trimmed, and sorted.

Benefits of licorice

Licorice has been given for digestive conditions such as peptic ulcers, heartburn, colic, food poisoning, and inflammation of the stomach lining. Traditionally, it has been prescribed for sore throat, bronchitis, tuberculosis, cough, and upper respiratory tract caused by bacteria and viruses. People with osteoarthritis, systemic lupus erythematosus (SLE), malaria, and chronic fatigue syndrome (CFS) have allegedly benefited from its healing properties. When applied topically, licorice is said to reduce the greasiness of hair.

It has been combined with other herbs. With Asian ginseng and Chinese thoroughwax, it can trigger the adrenal glands to function normally again, especially in people who have taken corticosteroids for a long time. When added as an ingredient in the shakuyaku-kanzo-to, it is believed to improve the fertility of women suffering from polycystic ovary syndrome. Other herbal combination with licorice claim to heal prostate cancer or eczema.

What to look out for

When consumed in amounts normally found in food, licorice is generally safe. If used in amounts generally contained in herbal medication for a limited period of time, licorice might be safe for use. When taking licorice longer than a month, it might cause harmful effects such as high blood pressure, low potassium levels in the blood, feebleness, paralysis, or worse, brain damage in otherwise healthy people. For those who consume large amounts of salt in their diet or have heart or kidney disease, and blood pressure, anything over five grams of licorice per day is lethal. It might also cause fatigue, headache, oedema, poor libido in men, or missed menstruation in women.

Pregnant women should never consume licorice as it might cause miscarriage or premature delivery. Not much data is known about its safety in breastfeeding women but to be safe, stay away from licorice. People with certain conditions should also be wary of using licorice as an herbal medication. It might worsen hypertensive episodes, increase the risk for intermittent heartbeats, exacerbate congestive heart failure, further impair people with potassium imbalance, and inflame hormone sensitive conditions such as certain cancers, uterine fibroids, or endometriosis. It can also make kidney diseases and men's libido go downhill.

Licorice can interact with a lot of medications, especially those that are used for heart diseases and hypertensive conditions. It can also interact with corticosteroids, diuretics, antidepressants, insulin or other hypoglycemic medications, birth control pills, and laxatives, even those that have to be metabolised by the liver such as celecoxib, fluvastatin, phenytoin, phenobarbital, and the like.

How to use licorice

Traditionally, licorice is taken as a tea. About one to four grams of powdered licorice root is steeped in 150 millilitres of boiling water to make a cup of tea taken thrice daily. For those who can withstand the taste, a dose of one to four grams of licorice root is given thrice daily. A ratio of one part licorice to five parts alcohol tincture may be given at two to five millilitres thrice daily.

For an upset stomach, an herbal combination that contains licorice is given at 20 drops every eight hours for a month. Alternatively, 760 to 1520 milligrams of licorice supplement may be chewed after meals for about two to four months to improve ulcers. To relieve coughs, 0.5 to a gram of powdered root may be taken every six to eight hours daily.

Topically, a two per cent licorice gel has been found to relieve the itching, swelling, and redness of people suffering from eczema. Some slimming gels also contain licorice for spot on fat reduction but more data is needed to prove its safety and effectiveness.

Studies on licorice

Licorice contains a variety of potent compounds. Glycyrrhizin, glycyrrhizic acid, glycyrrhizinate, liquiritin, and glabridin are some of the components currently studied for their properties.

When combined with other herbs such as peppermint leaves, German chamomile, caraway seeds, lemon balm, clown's mustard, celandine, angelica and milk thistle, licorice is found to be effective in reducing the frequency of heartburn. A dose that is taken for a month was able to reduce acid reflux and the pain, cramping, nausea, and vomiting that comes along with it.

Some data have been provided that licorice' demulcent effect might actually speed up the healing of stomach ulcers. There is also preliminary research that showed licorice and peony was able to reduce muscle cramps in people with liver disease and those who are undergoing hemodialysis. In a separate study, the chemicals in licorice have been able to demonstrate that it can be effective in treating hepatitis B and hepatitis C when given intravenously. However, there needs to be more subjects involved in the study in order to provide sufficient evidence for licorice' effectiveness for such conditions.

Conflicting evidence was presented on the claims that licorice can help manage weight. There is evidence that licorice extracts can reduce body fat. However, the herb also causes unavoidable water retention that any weight loss might not be noticeable at all. Other contradictory data also involved licorice effect in treating eczema.

References:

- Drugs.com. "Licorice professional information from Drugs.com." 2009. http://www.drugs.com/npp/licorice.html (accessed 14 Jun 2013).

- Medline Plus. "Licorice: MedlinePlus Supplements." 2012. http://www.nlm.nih.gov/medlineplus/druginfo/natural/881.html (accessed 14 Jun 2013).

- Medscape. "Licorice." 2013. http://reference.medscape.com/drug/alcacuz-chinese-licorice-licorice-344517 (accessed 14 Jun 2013).

• University of Maryland Medical Center. "Licorice." 2003. http://umm.edu/health/medical/altmed/herb/licorice (accessed 14 Jun 2013).

• WebMD. "LICORICE: Uses, Side Effects, Interactions and Warnings - WebMD." 2009. http://www.webmd.com/vitamins-supplements/ingredientmono-881-LICORICE.aspx?activeIngredientId=881&activeIngredientName=LIC ORICE (accessed 14 Jun 2013).

MA HUANG- Ma huang is a shrub native to China. Although ma huang is a collective term used by the Chinese for all other species of Ephedra, the most abundant is known by its scientific name Ephedra sinica but some people have called it ephedra, yellow horse, sea grape, herbal ecstasy, or desert herb. The whole plant is used for medicine and contains a potent chemical known as ephedrine, which has a variety of uses. Other species of ma huang known as American ephedra (Ephedra gerardiana) have been used by native Indian Americans for tea.

Growing ma huang

Ma huang is an evergreen shrub that can grow at about four feet high. The plant grows on sandy seashores and in temperate climates. It is almost leafless but it has thin, tube-like, yellowish green branches and runners underground. The leaves appear from December to January while the flowers bloom from May to June. The flowers produce fleshy cones that look like berries by August. For herbalists, the young stems and the small branches are the parts used for herbal medication. Compared to other related plants of the same genus, ma huang is rich in alkaloids that are chemically similar to amphetamines.

Ma huang is often grown from seeds as soon as it is ripe. It may be grown in spring or autumn, although inside a greenhouse in sandy compost. The seedlings are transplanted as soon as they're grown big enough until their first winter in the greenhouse. They can then be grown outside early summer on a well-drained loamy soil and under direct sunlight.

Benefits of ma huang

Because of its ephedrine content, ma huang has had a variety of benefits as an herbal medication. Extracts have been employed to manage obesity and enhance athletic performance. Some people have taken it for their respiratory allergies, nasal congestion, and flu. It has been given for fever, chills, headaches, aching of the bone and joints, and as a diuretic for those with oedema. Ma huang has been prescribed in traditional Chinese medicine for more than five millennia as a major treatment for asthma and bronchitis.

What to look out for

Ma huang is banned in the United States because of some safety issues since April 2004. It has also been banned by major athletic organisations as one of the doping supplements used by athletes to have an unfair advantage over their competitors.

Using ma huang can cause light-headedness, excitability, anxiety, very strong heartbeats, headache, poor appetite, nausea, and vomiting. However, there are more serious side effects that this herb is capable of. High blood pressure, heart attacks, seizures, strokes, irregular heartbeats, loss of consciousness, muscle disorders, and worse, death even in healthy people. These are seen in people who have been using abnormally high doses of ma huang or have been using them for a long time. It can also manifest when ma huang is combined with other stimulating herbs such as coffee, tea, kola nut, guarana, and mate.

People with certain conditions should not use ma huang. Pregnant and breastfeeding women should never use ma huang. Other medical conditions that should not be using ma huang or any of its extracts are angina, arrhythmia, anxiety, diabetes, essential tremors, hypertension, kidney stones, glaucoma, seizures, and pheochromocytoma.

Many medications interact with ma huang. Drugs that cause irregular heartbeats and stimulate the nervous system will definitely interact with this herb and will trigger a heart attack, a hypertensive crisis or make you more anxious than usual. Some medications to watch out for are amiodarone, disopyramide, quinidine, thioridazine, epinephrine, and many other similar drugs.

How to use ma huang

Ma huang is used differently in traditional Chinese medicine and Western medicine. There is no standard dose for ma huang but anything directed in the package labelling should be followed or at least under supervision of a healthcare professional. Standardised extracts are often sold as tinctures, tablets or capsules which might provide a dependable dose of the herb.

The recommended dose for ma huang is no more than 100 milligrams a day and no longer than two weeks. However, some people might find 100 milligrams a day is too high. The United States Food and Drug Administration (US FDA) has recommended that ma huang should be taken in doses not higher than eight milligrams per dose, and taken not more than every six hours, which should not exceed a total dose of 24 milligrams of ma huang per day.

Studies on ma huang

Ma huang contains alkaloids ephedrine and pseudoephedrine which stimulates the heart, the lungs, and the nervous system. The alkaloid was discovered by Chinese researchers in 1924 where Merck Pharmaceuticals eventually made synthetic versions of it two years after. Ephedrine is a salt that appears as shiny, white crystals that dissolve easily in water.

Its effects are similar to adrenaline, the body's biochemical stimulant for sympathetic nerves. Because of this, many manufacturers have claimed it for a variety of uses. Unfortunately, there is insufficient evidence for ma huang's effectiveness in improving athletic performance, keep allergies in check, clear nasal congestion, or even cool down fever.

There is compelling evidence that ma huang can be produce modest weight loss when combined with exercise and low fat diet. It was able to consistently produce a weight loss of 0.9 kilograms a month for about six months. It is not known whether it continues to produce weight loss beyond this period. When combined with other herbs such as cola nut and willow bark, ma huang can also cause similar weight loss.

A commercial supplement that contained ma huang, guarana, and other supplements were able to reduce weight by 2.7 kilograms per two months. Another combination of 90 milligrams of ma huang with 192 milligrams of cola nut was able to shed 5.3 kilograms in six months. However, the results also showed that it can produce devastating side effects, even in normally healthy people who follow the instructions carefully. The herb can cause small changes in blood pressure and heart rate.

References:

• National Center for Complementary and Alternative Medicine (NCCAM). "Ephedra | NCCAM." 2004. http://nccam.nih.gov/health/ephedra (accessed 14 Jun 2013).

• University of Maryland Medical Center. "Ephedra." 2004. http://umm.edu/health/medical/altmed/herb/ephedra (accessed 14 Jun 2013).

• WebMD. "EPHEDRA (Ma Huang): Uses, Side Effects, Interactions and Warnings - WebMD." 2009. http://www.webmd.com/vitamins-supplements/ingredientmono-847-ephedra.aspx?activeIngredientId=847&activeIngredientName=ephedra&source=1 (accessed 14 Jun 2013).

• Mayo Clinic. "Ephedra (Ephedra sinica) / ma huang - MayoClinic.com." 2012. http://www.mayoclinic.com/health/ephedra/NS_patient-ephedra (accessed 14 Jun 2013).

Drugs.com. "Ma huang medical facts from Drugs.com." 2010. http://www.drugs.com/mtm/ma-huang.html (accessed 14 Jun 2013).

MARSHMALLOW- Marshmallow is a plant whose leaves and roots produce copious mucilage that have been used as herbal medicine. Its scientific name is Althea officinalis and has been called by other common names such as sweet weed, wymote, mortification root, mallards, malvavisco, and guimauve.

Growing marshmallow

The marshmallow plant flourished originally in salt rich marsh soils, in damp meadows, beside ditches, by the sea shores, and the bans of tidal rivers. It has even adapted in moist, virgin soil. It is found growing in South and Western Europe, western Asia and the northeast part of North America.

The marshmallow is grown from its seeds which are sown in spring or through stem cuttings. Once the roots appear by autumn, they are carefully divided and replanted. They are grown at least two feet apart and thrive best in damp soil, usually near ditches and streams. The leaves are often picked in August before the flowers bloom.

Marshmallow has fleshy, straight stems that grow for about three to four feet. The leaves grow from short stems and have irregular, serrated margins. The stems and the leaves are covered with soft, downy fur. The flowers have five red tinted white petals. It has whitish yellow roots that are often long and narrow with a hardy but supple exterior. The whole plant is rich in tasteless mucilage.

Benefits of marshmallow

Marshmallow has been prescribed for any pain or swelling of the membranes lining the respiratory tract. It has benefited people suffering from dry cough, inflamed stomach lining, peptic ulcers, constipation, inflammation of the urinary tract, and even those with kidney stones. Marshmallow leaf and root have been applied directly on skin abscesses and ulcers and even as poultice for inflamed, burnt, insect bitten or wounded skin. It also acts as a flavouring ingredient in food.

What to look out for

Marshmallow is generally safe for most people who take it orally or when applied directly on the skin. For some people, it might cause a huge drop in blood sugar levels. This concern for marshmallow's ability to lower blood sugar extends to diabetics who are contemplating on using this herbal medication. Blood sugar levels should be monitored regularly to avoid dangerously low levels of blood sugar in the body.

If possible, marshmallow supplements must be stopped at least two weeks before a scheduled surgery or dental procedure so that it might not interfere with blood sugar management during and after the procedure.

Although there are little evidence of marshmallow safety on pregnant and breastfeeding women, the tea made of marshmallow have been used to stimulate the flow of breast milk. However, most supplements contain other herbs aside from marshmallow which might not be good for pregnant and nursing women. Check the label or go for whole marshmallow tea instead.

Some medications might interact with marshmallow. Aside from anti-diabetes medication which should be monitored or changed by your healthcare provider, it can also affect drugs that contain lithium. The plant has an inherent diuretic effect which can affect how fast the body can get rid of lithium from its circulation.

With marshmallow, lithium tends to stay longer in the body and might cause serious side effects in its wake. Its mucilage content might also affect how much drug your body can absorb orally. It can decrease the effectiveness of some medication. It can be avoided by taking marshmallow an hour after the medications have been taken by mouth.

How to use marshmallow

Marshmallow has often evoked images of the puffy confection but it is an actual plant. This variety has been used for more than two millennia as both food and medicine by the Romans, Chinese, Egyptians, and Syrians. The Arabs have been making its leaves into poultices for skin inflammation. The roots and leaves contain a mucilage that forms a slick gel when mixed with water.

Marshmallow has been eaten as an edible vegetable by the early Romans. Syrians will boil the roots and then sauté it with onions and butter, especially when food is scarce. The French eat the young tops and tender leaves raw by mixing it in their spring salad for its reputed stimulating effect on the kidneys. The English have used the mucilage for its confectionary paste which is an emollient which soothes cough and hoarseness. When cooked, the leaves can thicken the soup or as potherb.

The water used from boiling can substitute egg whites in making meringues. The teas are often made from flowers. The dried root is often given to teething children that helps soften the gum for erupting teeth and easing the pain associated with it. The mucilage has also been used on the skin to soften it. It can also be applied on open wounds, cuts, abrasions, and minor burns for immediate relief. An ointment containing marshmallow root mucilage is applied on boils and abscesses.

Dried marshmallow leaves have been used in poultices, tea, infusions, fluid extracts, and tinctures. The roots are often sold dried, either peeled or not and mixed as extracts, tinctures, capsules, syrups including those in ointments and creams. The dose for marshmallow is often dependent on the type of formulation it is in.

Studies on marshmallow

The root of the marshmallow is the richest source of mucilage at 25 to 35 per cent. Nevertheless, the amount of purified, mucilaginous polysaccharides is lower. The mucilage content is often dependent on the season, as it is most abundant in the winter. Standardised mucilage will contain rhamnose, galactose, galacturonic acid, and glucoronic acid. The root also contains asparagine, some sugars, pectin, and tannins. The flowers, leaves, and roots have also been found to contain glucosides.

Marshmallow is rich in mucilage that can form a protective lining on the skin and the digestive tract. It also has some active constituents that lessen coughing and heal wounds quickly. There is insufficient evidence of marshmallow's effectiveness to help conditions such as skin conditions, problems with bowel movement, peptic and intestinal ulcers, dry cough, and local irritation of the oral cavity.

References:

•   A Modern Herbal. "A Modern Herbal | Mallows." 2013. http://botanical.com/botanical/mgmh/m/mallow07.html (accessed 15 Jun 2013).

• Drugs.com. "Marsh Mallow professional information from Drugs.com." 2007. http://www.drugs.com/npp/marsh-mallow.html (accessed 15 Jun 2013).

• Plant Profiler. "Marshmallow (Althaea officinalis) | Plant Profiler." 2010. http://www.sigmaaldrich.com/life-science/nutrition-research/learning-center/plant-profiler/althaea-officinalis.html (accessed 15 Jun 2013).

• University of Maryland Medical Center. "Marshmallow." 2003. http://umm.edu/health/medical/altmed/herb/marshmallow (accessed 15 Jun 2013).

WebMD. "MARSHMALLOW: Uses, Side Effects, Interactions and Warnings - WebMD." 2009. http://www.webmd.com/vitamins-supplements/ingredientmono-774-MARSHMALLOW.aspx?activeIngredientId=774&activeIngredientName=MARSHMALLOW (accessed 15 Jun 2013).

MILK THISTLE- Milk thistle is a flowering herb that belongs to a group of thistles which have been considered as a weed. However, the Silybum marianum is a very valuable herbal medicine for conditions of the liver and gallbladder and its ability to reduce mortality from mushroom poisoning. It has been called by many names: bull thistle, Scotch thistle, blessed thistle, lady's milk, silibinin, and silymarin, The name comes from the milky sap that comes out of the leaves when it is crushed.

Growing milk thistle

Milk thistle is a native herb of the Mediterranean but now it has been cultivated all over the world. The plant spreads quickly and can be harvested in less than a year. It has been used for over two millennia as traditional cure for liver, kidney, and gallbladder disorders.

This type of thistle is the most medicinally valuable. It grows tall and slender with spiny stems branching at the top. It can grow to about five to 10 feet high. The wide leaves are waved and spiny at the margin with deep, shiny green accented with milky white veins. The flower heads are reddish purple and ridged with sharp spines. It blooms from June to August in the Northern Hemisphere or December to February in the Southern Hemisphere. It eventually bears small, brown spotted, shiny fruit that has a hard skin. The plant prefers to grow in dry, sunny areas.

Benefits of milk thistle

Traditionally, the milk thistle is believed to stimulate the flow of breast milk in nursing women. It has been prescribed for liver, spleen, and gallbladder conditions. Aside from expelling gallstones, it is also taken for dropsy. It also acts as a demulcent for those suffering from inflamed lining of the lungs and viscous phlegm. The young, tender plant when eaten is a reputed blood cleanser. Some people claim that milk thistle can lower levels of bad cholesterol in the circulation, reduce growth of certain cancers such as breast, cervical, and prostate.

What to look out for

Milk thistle is generally safe for a majority of people. Many studies have shown it can be used safely for up to 41 months. However, it might have a laxative effect. Other less common side effects reported are nausea, indigestion, gas, bloating, and poor appetite.

Taking milk thistle might also trigger allergic reactions in people who are also allergic to ragweed, marigolds, daisies, and other similar plants. People with oestrogen-sensitive conditions should also be wary of milk thistle as it can worsen endometriosis, uterine fibroids, as well as cancers of the breast, uterus, and ovaries.

Because milk thistle can interact with the liver, many medications can interact with it. Medication that need to be metabolised by the liver such as diazepam, celecoxib, irbesartan, phenytoin, tamoxifen, torsemide, ketoconazole, fexodenadine, and similar medications might have an increased effect and at the same time, increases the risk for side effects. Oestrogen containing medications such as estradiol, birth control pills, and the like will decrease its effects. In addition, cholesterol lowering medications such as atorvastatin, lovastatin, rosuvastatin and the like might have erratic effects when given with milk thistle.

How to use milk thistle

The stalks of the milk thistle are edible, aside from being palatable and nutrient rich. The young leaves may also be eaten in salads. The young shoots cut close to the roots along with some parts of the stalk may be boiled and is comparable in taste to cabbage or baked in pies. The roots are eaten similar to salsify or roasted and used as a substitute for coffee.

Products containing milk thistle should have about 70 to 80 per cent of silymarin. These are often made from seeds. Commercially prepared supplements with milk thistle are sold as tinctures, liquid extracts, or capsules containing 120 to 140 milligrams of silymarin. Newer preparations may contain a complex made of phosphatidylcholine as it is easily absorbed by the body. Phosphatidylcholine helps silymarin attach to cell membrane with ease and keep toxins out of cells, especially that of the liver. Supplements containing only silibinin are given at 240 milligrams twice daily for chronic active hepatitis. A dose of 200 milligrams of silymarin every eight hours is given for diabetes.

There is no standard dose when using milk thistle as a supplement. However, there are some doses that have been used in scientific research. A thistle extracts containing 140 milligrams of silymarin is given every eight hours for allergic rhinitis. For mild to moderate cases of dyspepsia, there is a supplement that contains milk thistle in combination with other herbs which may be given at a dose of 20 drops thrice daily. In clinical trials, a dose of 13 grams of silibinin is usually given in divided doses for mushroom poisoning. It has also been given in children at a dose of 5.1 milligrams of silibinin for every kilogram weight per day.

Studies on milk thistle

Milk thistle seeds have been studied for its potential to protect liver cells from toxic chemicals and medications. It has potent antioxidant and anti-inflammatory effect. Milk thistle is a plant that has oestrogen-like effects. Silymarin is the principal active ingredient of milk thistle. Chemically, silymarin is a group of flavonoids that is made up of silibinin, silidianin, silidianin, silichristin and taxifolin.

Milk thistle has been found to be effective in lowering blood sugar in people with type II diabetes. When combined with other herbs, it can relieve dyspepsia. There are data that show milk thistle supplements as beneficial for people suffering from chronic liver disease caused by viral infections or alcohol abuse and cirrhosis. There is potential for milk thistle's use for diabetes and liver damage caused by other drugs or toxins in humans but there is very little data to support that.

However, there is insufficient evidence if milk thistle is really effective for conditions of the gallbladder or spleen. There is also very little data available regarding its effectiveness for swollen lungs, malaria, menstrual problems, and as an antidote for mushroom poisoning.

References:

• Drugs.com. "Milk Thistle professional information from Drugs.com." 2010. http://www.drugs.com/npp/milk-thistle.html (accessed 15 Jun 2013).

• Mayo Clinic. "Milk thistle (Silybum marianum) - MayoClinic.com." 2012. http://www.mayoclinic.com/health/silymarin/NS_patient-milkthistle (accessed 15 Jun 2013).

• Medscape. "Medscape: Medscape Access." 2013. http://reference.medscape.com/drug/carduus-marianum-holy-thistle-milk-thistle-344521 (accessed 15 Jun 2013).

• National Center for Complementary and Alternative Medicine (NCCAM). "Milk Thistle | NCCAM." 2012. http://nccam.nih.gov/health/milkthistle/ataglance.htm (accessed 15 Jun 2013).

University of Maryland Medical Center. "Milk thistle." 2006. http://umm.edu/health/medical/altmed/herb/milk-thistle (accessed 15 Jun 2013).

MULLEIN- Mullein is a hairy wildflower that is known for its antimicrobial, expectorant, analgesic, and moisturising properties. Its scientific name is mullein Verbascum thapsus and is sometimes referred to as common mullein. It has also been called by other names such as candle flower and beggar's blanket.

Growing mullein

Mullein is a plant native to Europe as well as northern parts of Africa and Asia. The herb has been introduced in the Americas and Australia. It's a hardy plant that can grow on a variety of soils but it flourishes best on soils with the full sun. It has been considered as a weed by some countries as it spreads fast through its prolific seeds. It is not cultivated.

Mullein has small, yellow flowers that are clumped on a tall stem which is surrounded by a rosette of leaves at its base. The bluish-green rosette appears in its first year of growth and the year after, the single straight stem appears. The five-petal flowers are arranged alternately along the stems. It blooms from June to September. It eventually produces a capsule which contains numerous brown seeds. These seeds are very fertile and can be stored for years.

Benefits of mullein

Mullein is a folk remedy for any condition associated with coughs, pains, and skin problems. It is given for whooping cough, tuberculosis, bronchitis, pneumonia, flu, allergies, asthma, colds, and sore throat. Agonising ailments such as earaches, tonsillitis, colic, migraine, rheumatism, and gout seem to benefit from mullein. It has also been applied for wounds, burns, haemorrhoids, bruises, and infections of the skin to heal and protect it. Other people have utilised mullein preparations as a sedative and a diuretic.

What to look out for

No side effects or toxic reactions have been identified in using mullein as an herbal medication. However, pregnant and breastfeeding women are advised to keep away from this herb until safety is established. The Food and Drugs Administration (FDA) has classified mullein as GRAS or generally recognised as safe.

Mullein seeds contain rotenone, a toxic chemical. It has been used as fish poison by those who fish using spears. For people using fresh mullein, make sure that there are no seeds present on the flowers. A safer alternative is to use leaves. When using mullein oil should check first whether their eardrums are perforated or not before using the product.

How to use mullein

The flowers, leaves, and root of the mullein have been used for herbal medicine. These yellow flowers have been used as hair dye. The roots were often boiled and given for croup or colds. The leaves were applied on the skin to keep it soft and protected. Oil made from flowers is made by macerating the flowers in olive oil inside a sealed bottle and placed near the fire or exposed to the sun for 21 days which can be applied on earaches, eczema, and frostbitten skin. Various preparations have been made of mullein. It has been consumed, applied locally on the skin, or even smoked.

There is no standard dose for mullein supplements but the usual dose is given at three to four grams a day, sometimes in divided doses. Mullein tea is made by adding a teaspoon or two of dried flowers and leaves to a cup of boiling water. It is steeped for 10 minutes and drained before drinking. The tea can be consumed regularly as it is rich in B vitamins, choline, hesperidin, and minerals like magnesium and sulphur. An alcoholic tincture of fresh mullein is given at eight to 10 drops in cold water for migraine or chronic headaches. It might be a bit bitter than the tea but it's free from irritating hairs from the leaves. The long taproot can be used for problems in the urinary tract.

Pre-packed mullein oil for earaches should be brought at room temperature before dripping into the ear canal. The oil has also been used for sores, eczema, boils, and chilblains. A poultice of leaves has been used for haemorrhoids. Flower preserves have been employed for ringworm while a root infusion has been used for athlete's foot. Rubbing warts with mullein juice or powdered dried roots are believed to be effective. A wash made from flowers can be used as a disinfectant for small wounds and abrasions.

Native American Indians have smoked the leaves for pulmonary conditions. The leaves are dried and blended with other herbs such as coltsfoot or jimsonweed.

Studies on mullein

The mucilaginous herb is bitter and cooling which has been used to sooth tissues. It is rich in saponins, mucilage, iridoid glycosides, flavonoids, and phenolic acids. Verbascosaponin, aucubin, and catalpol are some of the active ingredients identified in mullein. The mucilage helps loosen phlegm and soothe mucus membranes. Iridoid glycosides have been identified to fight inflammation. The flowers contain gum, resins, yellow and green dyes, fats, glucosides, some sugar, and a trace of minerals. The green part of the mullein is believed to contain some coumarin derivatives which might have an anticoagulant effect.

Mullein contains substances that are antiviral and antibacterial in respiratory conditions. When extracts are scrutinised, it has shown to kill viruses on contact, a property that might be useful for people suffering from flu. However, the research is quite limited to prove that it can fight viral infections in general.

There are double blind trials that involved children suffering from middle ear infection which studied the effect of standard earache anaesthetic made of ametocaine and phenazone compared to an herbal mix of mullein, garlic, St. John's wort, and calendula. The data showed both were equally effective in managing pain. The study has been criticised for the absence of a placebo group so more study is needed to validate its results.

There is very little data that can show mullein's effectiveness for the conditions it is traditionally used for. Anecdotal evidence has demonstrated that combining mullein with herbs of similar properties, such as yerba santa, marshmallow, elecampane, or cherry, is more effective than taken alone.

References:

• A Modern Herbal. "A Modern Herbal | Mullein, Great." 2005. http://botanical.com/botanical/mgmh/m/mulgre63.html (accessed 16 Jun 2013).

• Drugs.com. "Mullein information from Drugs.com." 2005. http://www.drugs.com/npc/mullein.html (accessed 16 Jun 2013).

• Health Library by iHerb. "Health Library - C573 - Mullein - Natural, Alternative - 21821." 1993. http://healthlibrary.epnet.com/GetContent.aspx?token=e0498803-7f62-4563-8d47-5fe33da65dd4&chunkiid=21821 (accessed 16 Jun 2013).

•   RxList. "Mullein Effectiveness, Safety, and Drug Interactions on RxList." 2013. http://www.rxlist.com/mullein/supplements.htm (accessed 16 Jun 2013).

•   WebMD. "MULLEIN: Uses, Side Effects, Interactions and Warnings - WebMD." 2009. http://www.webmd.com/vitamins-supplements/ingredientmono-572-MULLEIN.aspx?activeIngredientId=572&activeIngredientName=MULLEIN (accessed 16 Jun 2013).

MYRRH- Myrrh is a resin of small, thorny trees related to the frankincense or it might also refer to an unrelated herb known as cicely, with scientific name Myrrhis odorata. However, myrrh resin is a valuable herbal medicine that has been worth its weight in gold since ancient times.

Myrrh oleoresin comes from a cut through the bark that penetrates the sapwood. It is usually harvested from Commiphora myrrha that is also known as African myrrh, myrrh gum, mo yao, opopanax, bol, and didin. The term comes from Aramaic "murr" which meant bitter. Traditionally, it's used as incense and perfume.

Growing myrrh

The small, spiky trees where myrrh comes from can grow up to about three metres in height and is indigenous to Africa, the eastern Mediterranean, and south Arabia. Myrrh comes from natural cracks on the trunk or on artificial fissures made to harvest it. It is often harvested during the summer and the oil is often extracted through steam distillation. The trees where myrrh is harvested have knotted branches that have smaller branches at right angles with terminal spikes. Its leaves are trifoliate but small and oval shaped. The flowers are small and white.

Benefits of myrrh

Myrrh has been utilised by traditional Chinese medicine for its supposedly beneficial effects to the meridians of the heart, liver, and spleen in addition to its ability to stimulate stagnant circulation in the uterus. It has been recommended for rheumatism, arthritis, circulatory conditions, and gynaecological problems. Middle Eastern medicine have given it for wounds and infections. Ayurvedic and Unani medicine has long incorporated myrrh for its tonic and rejuvenating properties. Western medicine has long recognised myrrh's antiseptic and analgesic properties.

Myrrh benefits people who suffer from dyspepsia, stomach ulcers, arthritis, and respiratory problems such as colds, cough, or asthma. Some have claimed it is also an effective stimulant for menstrual flow and even conditions such as leprosy, syphilis, and cancer. Topically, it can relieve all sorts of mouth problems that is characterised by pain and swelling. It has also been applied on haemorrhoids, bedsores, boils, wounds, and scrapes.

What to look out for

When used in small amount, myrrh seems to be safe for most people. When applied directly on the skin, it might trigger rash formation or diarrhoea if ingested. Doses higher than two to four grams have caused kidney irritation and problems with irregular heart rates.

Myrrh is not safe for pregnant women as it can stimulate the uterus and cause miscarriage. Although there is no data regarding myrrh's safety for nursing women, stay on the safe side and avoid use. Women suffering from uterine bleeding should stay clear of using this supplement as it might worsen the bleeding. It can also interact with warfarin effectiveness, which can increase the risk of bleeding.

Diabetic patients should also be wary of its property of lowering levels of blood sugar. Monitor blood sugar levels when using myrrh with anti-diabetic medications. This is also a major concern for those who have a scheduled surgery and medical or dental procedure. Stop using myrrh two weeks before the appointed surgery or procedure. Anti-diabetic drugs such as glyburide, insulin, pioglitazone, tolbutamide, and the like will drop blood sugar to dangerously low levels.

People with heart problems and systemic inflammation should not use myrrh. In large amounts, myrrh might make the conditions worse.

How to use myrrh

Tinctures made of myrrh are not diluted. These are often painted or dabbed on the affected areas twice to thrice a day. Mouth rinses may be given at five to 10 drops in a glass of water while gargles use about 1.5 to 3 millilitres of the tincture in a glass of water. Dental powders are often standardised to contain 10 per cent of the resin.

Teas made of myrrh are given at a teaspoon or two of the powdered resin for every cup of boiling water. It is steeped for 10 to 15 minutes and drank every eight hours. Alternatively, a typical dose of one gram of myrrh is ingested thrice daily.

The European Medicines Agency has recognised the traditional use of myrrh as treatment for mouth ulcers and gum infections and for the treatment of small wounds and boils. All of these indications refer to myrrh's antiseptic and astringent property. In the United States, myrrh is recognised as a natural flavouring substance for food and the tincture as an astringent in oral health products.

Studies on myrrh

Myrrh gum is a sap that comes out of the trees which may appear like clear, yellow wax that eventually coagulates and become hard and glossy with streaks of white the longer it is stored. Its volatile oil contains sesquiterpenes, sterols, and steroids. The gum part of the resin is abundant in polysaccharides and proteins. Its furanosesquiterpenes have been identified for myrrh's characteristic odour as well as its antiseptic and hypoglycemic effects. There are two other sesquiterpenes that have been able to demonstrate its activity on opioid receptors of the nervous system, which validates its analgesic effect.

Myrrh may be a potential agent for the management and treatment of schistosomiasis and fascioliasis. However, more studies are underway to prove its apparent effects on the infestations. Human subjects infected with various schistosomes have shown that myrrh has been able to eliminate the parasites to the liver where they eventually underwent phagocytosis. The similar mechanism has also been observed for those affected with fascioliasis. However, large scale studies have yet to show its effectiveness for this infestation.

Another clinical study involved the comparison of herbal toothpaste with myrrh and conventional commercial toothpaste. Based on the randomised, double-blind controlled study, the herbal toothpaste containing myrrh was just as effective as ordinary toothpaste in keeping gingival and periodontal infections in check.

Most of the studies done on myrrh for its alleged potency and indications have involved mostly animal subjects. Other data on its effects on humans are mostly based on case reports and in vitro studies which are limited and needs to be further investigated.

References:

• A Modern Herbal. "A Modern Herbal | Myrrh." 2010. http://botanical.com/botanical/mgmh/m/myrrh-66.html (accessed 16 Jun 2013).

• Drugs.com. "Myrrh professional information from Drugs.com." 2008. http://www.drugs.com/npp/myrrh.html (accessed 16 Jun 2013).

• Discovery Fit and Health. "Discovery Health "Myrrh: Herbal Remedies"." 2009. http://health.howstuffworks.com/wellness/natural-medicine/herbal-remedies/myrrh-herbal-remedies.htm (accessed 16 Jun 2013).

• RxList. "Myrrh Effectiveness, Safety, and Drug Interactions on RxList." 2013. http://www.rxlist.com/myrrh/supplements.htm (accessed 16 Jun 2013).

• WebMD. "Myrrh: Uses, Side Effects, Interactions and Warnings - WebMD." 2007. http://www.webmd.com/vitamins-supplements/ingredientmono-570-myrrh.aspx?activeIngredientId=570&activeIngredientName=myrrh (accessed 16 Jun 2013).

NETTLE- Nettle is a collective term for the plants of the genus Urtica. The most popular of all nettles in this group is the common nettle, also known by its scientific name Urtica dioica. The common nettle has also been called stinging nettle, gerrais, isirgan, kazink, and devil's leaf. This plant is notorious for its stinging hairy leaves and stems that inject chemicals such as histamine, serotonin, and choline to produce a stinging sensation upon contact. Despite its infamy, the nettle has been used both as food and medicine.

Growing nettle

The common nettle is found in the temperate areas of Europe and Asia as well as some areas in South Africa, Canada, Australia, and the Andes.

Nettle has a heart-shaped, finely toothed, dark green leaves that have a tapered tip. It has green flowers growing in long, branched clusters and will appear different, depending on their gender. The flowers bloom from June to September. Nettle fruits appear as small, oval-shaped seeds that are small and somewhat tan in color. The stems will often grow from two to three feet. The roots are creeping and very prolific, making nettle widespread and difficult to control. The whole plant is covered with stinging hairs

Benefits of nettle

Traditionally, nettle has been employed as an adjuvant for arthritis. Native American have utilised nettle tea to ease labour and to help stimulate the flow of breast milk in nursing women. Its irritating effects have provided temporary relief from rheumatism. Nettle juice has been given for insect bites and stings. European herbalists have prescribed nettle tea for disorders of the lungs.

Modern herbalists have recognised the benefit of nettle root extract for those with enlarged prostate and for removing stones in the urinary tract. It is an effective diuretic and has also been given for swollen joints and prostate, hypertension, and allergic rhinitis.

Nettle extracts have also been applied as natural anti-dandruff, an herbal treatment for baldness, and to keep hair from being too greasy.

What to look out for

In general, nettle leaves have been generally safe because it has been used for a long time. Nettle roots have undergone safety studies in Germany and no adverse reactions have been reported. There has been concern because nettle might interact with medications that have been prescribed for diabetes, hypertension, inflammation, and sedation. However, there has yet to be determined.

There are concerns that nettle extracts might affect pregnant and nursing women because it has been used for inducing abortions. Nevertheless, many cultures have employed nettle leaf tea for these women.

How to use nettle

The common nettle has been eaten as food. Its taste has been compared to that of spinach and cucumber. It is rich in vitamins A and C as well as minerals such as iron, potassium, manganese and calcium. The tops have been harvested by Native American Indians as vegetable when food is scarce. It has been used as soups in Europe and has been cooked with spices in India.

Dosage of nettles is variable and highly dependent on label instructions. Some commercial preparations with nettle root have standardised scopoletin content, although it has yet to be recognised as an active ingredient. Nettle infusions have been used for anaemia, heavy menstruation, and skin complaints.

The juice of the nettle roots or leaves is mixed with honey or sugar for asthmatics. Dried nettle leaves can be burnt and inhaled to have the same bronchodilating effect. Nettle root tea may be given for those who suffer from oedema or as a mild diuretic. The seeds and flowers are steeped in wine for fevers. The powdered seeds are given for goitre and to reduce weight. Consuming nettle seeds are used as antidotes for hemlock, henbane, and nightshade poisoning.

Young nettle tops are simmered in a quart of water for two hours and eventually strained and bottled when cold. This preparation is often applied topically for healthy scalp. Another alternative is to boil the whole plant in vinegar and water and straining it before use. To stimulate hair follicle growth, juice of nettles is used.

For allergies such as hay fever, a dose of 300 milligrams of lyophilised nettle leaf given twice daily is found effective. For BPH, 360 milligrams of aqueous extracts of nettle root is given daily in divided doses for six months. Alternatively, 600 to 1,200 milligrams of alcohol-based nettle root extract is given every day for six to nine weeks for BPH. According to most manufacturers, nettle supplements must be taken for a month before its effects can be evident.

Studies on nettle

Formic acid, mucilage, mineral salts, ammonia, and carbonic acid have been found in fresh nettles. The formic acid, its phosphate content, and the hint of iron have made nettle a valuable food medicine.

There are studies in the late 90's that have studied the common nettle's ability to inhibit inflammatory chemicals such as cytokines. According to their data, nettle leaf flowers have been able to lower the levels of Tumour Necrotic Factor (TNF) alpha. It does this by preventing the transcription factor in genes that activate its production in the synovial lining of the joints. It has shown potential for management of inflamed joints.

Nettle root extracts have undergone clinical studies for its beneficial effects on the symptoms of benign prostatic hyperplasia (BPH). The extracts have shown to be better than the placebo even when given alone or in combination with other herbs.   Freeze dried nettle leaf extracts have shown some potential as treatment for hay fever, according to a preliminary double-blind study. There is also a small double-blind study that applied nettle leaves to painful joints and have shown to relieve symptoms.

The safety of nettle extracts has been studied for its side effects. The study involved more than 4,000 people who took 600 to 1,200 milligrams of nettle root extract every day for about half a year. Less than one per cent has complained of gastrointestinal upset while about 0.19 per cent had an outbreak of skin rash.

References:

- Drugs.com. "Nettles professional information from Drugs.com." 2010. http://www.drugs.com/npp/nettles.html (accessed 17 Jun 2013).

- Medscape. "Nettle." 2013. http://reference.medscape.com/drug/stinging-nettle-urtica-dioica-nettle-344572 (accessed 17 Jun 2013).

- RxList. "Stinging Nettle Effectiveness, Safety, and Drug Interactions on RxList." 2013. http://www.rxlist.com/stinging_nettle/supplements.htm (accessed 17 Jun 2013).

- University of Maryland Medical Center. "Stinging nettle." 2010. http://umm.edu/health/medical/altmed/herb/stinging-nettle (accessed 17 Jun 2013).

- WebMD. "STINGING NETTLE: Uses, Side Effects, Interactions and Warnings - WebMD." 2009. http://www.webmd.com/vitamins-supplements/ingredientmono-664-STINGING%20NETTLE.aspx?activeIngredientId=664&active IngredientName=STINGING%20NETTLE (accessed 17 Jun 2013).

PASSION FLOWER- Passion flower is a flourishing vine of the familiar, resilient wildflower of south eastern United States. Its scientific name is Passiflora incarnata and has been called by its other common names such as passion vine, may pop, water lemon, wild apricot, and wild passion vine. In other languages, it is referred to as fleishfarbige, maracuja, and corona de Cristo.

Growing passion flower

Passion flower was found while Spanish colonizers foraged in Peru in 1569. They thought the physical appearance of the flowers resembled the passion of Christ and that it was a go signal from above to take over the country. Passion flowers have been thought to show certain features of Jesus' crucifixion.

Meanwhile, the natives of Peru have already been using the plant as a calming sedative and mild analgesic. Europeans eventually used it as folk remedy and digestive aid. The extracts have been prescribed for anxiety and nervousness.

The stems of the passion flower are smooth, long, and trailing with lots of tendrils. The leaves are palm like and have lobed margins with glands at the base of the leaf's blade. Its flowers have five bluish-white petals with a ring of purple and white between its petals and stamens. It often blooms in July. The passion flower has a fleshy berry, known to some people as maypop, which is about the size of a chicken egg. Initially it appears green and turns orange as it ripens. Its yellow pulp is sweet and edible.

Benefits of passion flower

Whether fresh or dried, passion flower is a popular herbal medicine for managing anxiety and insomnia. The extract is believed to improve the quality of sleep. It has also been given for people suffering from poor digestion because of fretfulness or nervousness. It has also shown potential for managing symptoms related to narcotic withdrawal.

Although passion flower's popular indication is mostly for its sedative benefits, some people have taken it for other related conditions. Seizures, panic attacks, attention deficit-hyperactivity disorder (ADHD), jumpiness, irritability, tremors, and irregular heartbeats have benefited from its use. It has also been given for asthma, fibromyalgia, hypertension, and for relieving symptoms of menopause and muscle pain. Passion flower has also been applied locally to haemorrhoids, burns, and local swelling.

What to look out for

When taken in amounts typically found within food, passion flower is generally safe. It might be nontoxic if used for less than a month. When taken in significant amounts found in medicine, passion flower is not safe. It should never be given to pregnant women because it might stimulate the uterus and cause miscarriage. The chemicals found in passion flower might also intensify the expected effects of anaesthesia and other similar medicines that can produce sedating effects. Stop taking passion flower for at least two weeks before any scheduled surgery, dental or medical procedure.

People have reported side effects when using passion flower extracts. Light headedness, disorientation, irregularly fast heartbeats, poor muscle coordination and engorged blood vessels are some of the side effects commonly experienced by people taking the herb. Other people also reported feeling queasy, sleepy, and have irregular heart rate and rhythm.

Passion flower can also interact with other drugs and herbal supplements. It might increase the potency of medications that can depress the nervous system. With phenobarbital, clonazepam, zolpidem, and other similar drugs, passion flower might cause unusual excessive sleepiness. Herbs such as calamus, hops, catnip, kava, valerian, Californian poppy, skullcap, St. Johns wort, and other similar plants can also cause similar overly sedative effects when combined with the herb.

Passion flower has been sold over the counter since it's approval to be sold to consumers as a herbal sleep aid and a herbal sedative in the United States. However, the product has been withdrawn because there isn't enough evidence of its effectiveness and safety. It is still listed in the United States Food and Drug Administration (US FDA) as Generally Recognised as Safe (GRAS).

How to use passion flower

Passion flower has been combined with other herbs such as hops, valerian, skullcap, , kava and German chamomile as an herbal sedative. In 1985, Germany's Commission E officially approved passion flower's use as treatment for nervous problems.

Traditional use of passion flower is by taking a cup of tea thrice daily. The tea is made by steeping a tablespoon of dried leaves in a cup of boiling water for 10 to 15 minutes. For anxiety disorders, passion flower liquid extract is given at 15 drops thrice a day. Tablet formulation containing passion flower is given at 30 milligrams every eight hours. For muscle tensions, a dose of 30 to 60 liquid extract drops is given twice a day or up to every three hours, depending on the body's response. If using liquid passion flower extract for managing narcotic associated symptoms withdrawal, a dose of 15 drops is given with 0.2 milligrams of clonidine every six hours. Typical dose range from four to eight grams but is not recommended.

Studies on passion flower

The active ingredient in passion flower is not yet known. The alkaloids harman and harmaline found in its extracts have been found to have similar properties as the body's monoamine oxidase inhibitors and can also stimulate uterine contractions. It is not known if the whole plant has this property as well. Another component known as passiflorine have been compared to effects seen in morphine.

A month long double-blind study involved 36 anxious subjects have been studied. It aims to compare passion flower's effects to medical protocol oxazepam. What the data revealed was that oxazepam's effects were observed at a shorter period of time but in the end, passion flower is just as effective. Although its effects might take some time to manifest, the herb has a major advantage over oxazepam as it does not cause side effects that affect the subject's performance at work.

Another double-blind trial enlisted 65 men dependent on opiates. The study involved comparing the effect of passion flower with clonidine against clonidine alone. Clonidine has been given for narcotic withdrawal but it cannot control the emotional symptoms such as drug cravings, anxiety, irritability, and depression. At the end of the study, using passion flower and clonidine were able to ease these symptoms compared to clonidine alone.

References:

- A Modern Herbal. "A Modern Herbal | Passion Flower." 2009. http://botanical.com/botanical/mgmh/p/pasflo14.html (accessed 17 Jun 2013).

- Drugs.com. "Passion Flower professional information from Drugs.com." 2006. http://www.drugs.com/npp/passion-flower.html (accessed 17 Jun 2013).

- Medscape. "Medscape: Passion flower." 2013. http://reference.medscape.com/drug/apricot-vine-corona-de-cristo-passion-flower-344546 (accessed 17 Jun 2013).

- University of Maryland Medical Center. "Passionflower." 2001. http://umm.edu/health/medical/altmed/herb/passionflower (accessed 17 Jun 2013).

WebMD. "passionflower: Uses, Side Effects, Interactions and Warnings - WebMD." 2009. http://www.webmd.com/vitamins-supplements/ingredientmono-871-passionflower.aspx?activeIngredientId=871&activeIngredientName=passionflower (accessed 17 Jun 2013).

PEPPERMINT- Peppermint is a type of minty herb native to Europe. It is a member of the mint family that has been cultivated for its volatile oil which has been used as flavouring and herbal medicine. Its scientific name is Mentha piperita. It has been called bo he, menthe verte, and sentebon.

Growing peppermint

Peppermint is a hybrid made by crossing watermint and spearmint. It often grows in moist and damp places which are often undisturbed. It has been used by the Greeks and Romans for their sauces and wines. The Egyptians have cultivated it and have been found in pharmacopoeia of Iceland in the 13th century. Western Europe has used it as a herbal remedy in the 18th century.

Peppermint leaves are short with conspicuous stalks that are about two inches in length and about 0.75 to 1.5 inches wide. The leaf margins are serrated but it has a smooth surface. There is slight fuzz on the main veins ad midribs on the underside. Its purple green stems can be about two to four feet high. Peppermint flowers are often reddish violet and whorled clusters on the axils of the upper ends of the leaves. It does not bear any seeds. The whole plant has a characteristic smell caused by the volatile oil found in its parts.

Peppermint plants flourish in warm, moist, and rich soils than can retain moisture and drainage. Runners of the plant are often dug up in early spring, usually in April and May then placed in shallow troughs of rich soil. It is continuously weeded and nourished until it blooms in summer. When it has reached a height of about four inches, they are transferred to new plots until it grows on its own, branching stolons and runners about. It is then harvested by hand and distilled in straw while the stolons are ploughed in and fertilised before winter sets in.

Benefits of peppermint

Peppermint is a certified anti-spasmodic which relieves pains caused by spasms of the digestive tract. It has been prescribed for irritable bowel syndrome (IBS) and improves the movement of bile in the body. The menthol component of the herb has been used for respiratory conditions for its decongesting effect. It is also applied on the skin for its cooling and warming action to relieve pain. It has also be given for painful menstruation, sore throat, and inflamed oral cavity.

What to look out for

When used as seasoning or flavouring, peppermint is classified as generally recognised as safe (GRAS). However, when used as herbal remedy, peppermint can cause adverse reactions. However, the peppermint oil has been banned as an over-the-counter digestive aid in 1990 because its effectiveness has not been proven. Today, peppermint is sold as a dietary supplement.

People with gastro-oesophageal reflux disease (GERD) or even with active gastric ulcers should avoid peppermint oil because it might lower the pressure of the oesophageal sphincter. It should never be applied directly on the face, especially under the nose of a child or infant. Children older than eight years old may be given peppermint as it is likely safe. It can cause allergies such as reddening, headaches, and dermatitis. Pregnant women must not use it because of its reported emmenagogue effects and might trigger a miscarriage or premature birth.

Peppermint oil might interact with drug metabolism, especially those that pass through the liver, such as felodipine and simvastatin. Caffeine absorption may also be decreased while the effects of cyclosporine may also be decreased in people taking peppermint tea.

How to use peppermint

Peppermint oils have been given at 0.1 to 0.24 millilitres for its carminative effect. A combination of 90 milligrams peppermint oil with caraway oil has been given for stomach upset. Doses up to 1.2 grams daily have been placed in enteric-coated tablets for IBS. Peppermint oil might come with other herbs such as clown's mustard, German chamomile, caraway, liquorice, milk thistle, angelica, celandine, and lemon balm to relieve acid reflux, stomach cramps, nausea, and vomiting. About 40 millilitres of peppermint oil may also be mixed with barium suspensions used during colonoscopy. An inhaled dose of 0.2 millilitres peppermint mixed in two millilitres saline can be used to manage or prevent post-operative nausea. Peppermint oil can also be applied locally for tension headaches every 15 to 30 minutes.

Studies on peppermint

Peppermint oil is colourless, somewhat yellowish green with a pungent, penetrating odour and stinging, somewhat camphor taste. It eventually turns ruddy with age but takes on an improved fullness. The main component of the oil is menthol but it also contains menthyl acetate, menthone, cineol, pinene, and limonene. Its minty odour comes from the ester menthyl acetate but its medicinal value comes from its alcohol component, menthol.

There are studies done in uncovering peppermint's therapeutic properties in the digestive system. Animal studies have shown peppermint's ability to lessen the incidence of nausea. In humans, using menthol and peppermint oil are also effective in staving off nausea but are not as effective as standard medication. Another study showed peppermint oil alone or when combined with other herbs were able to perform better than the placebo in managing indigestion. In a separate study, peppermint oil's mechanism has been studied in slowing down spasms of the smooth muscle. According to their data, peppermint was able to exert its antispasmodic effect by blocking calcium channel pumps in the cell.

Aside from being a valuable herbal remedy for the digestive tract, researchers have also looked into peppermint's antitussive effect on children when inhaled. Menthol inhalation has also shown a decongesting effect although the mechanisms have yet to be determined. Explaining the sensory effect of peppermint has also been a subject of a separate study. According to this study, menthol has a cooling effect at low concentrations and at higher doses exerts a numbing, irritating effect. This is due to menthol's direct effect on the cold receptor which senses pain and temperature. When menthol binds to this receptor, it releases calcium and its sensory effects manifest.

References:

- Healthline. "What is Peppermint? Dosing, Side Effects & More." 2005. http://www.healthline.com/natstandardcontent/peppermint (accessed 18 Jun 2013).

- Patient.co.UK. "Peppermint oil | Medicine | Patient.co.uk." 2010. http://www.patient.co.uk/medicine/Peppermint-oil.htm (accessed 18 Jun 2013).

- WebMD. "Peppermint Oil: Uses, Side Effects, Interactions, Pictures, Warnings & Dosing." 2009. http://drugs.webmd.boots.com/drugs/drug-358-PEPPERMINT+OIL.aspx?drugid=358&drugname=PEPPERM

INT%2BOIL&source=2&isTicTac=false (accessed 18 Jun 2013).

- World's Healthiest Foods. "Peppermint." 2003. http://www.whfoods.com/genpage.php?tname=foodspice& dbid=102 (accessed 18 Jun 2013).

- Discovery Fit and Health. "Discovery Health "Peppermint: Herbal Remedies"." 2013. http://health.howstuffworks.com/wellness/natural-medicine/herbal-remedies/peppermint-herbal-remedies.htm (accessed 18 Jun 2013).

PSYLLIUM- Psyllium is a collective term for herbal plants that belong to the genus Plantago. Psyllium seeds have been used for their mucilage. Plantago psyllium and Plantago ovata are the major sources of psyllium fibre. The black seeds of the P. psyllium are also called fleaseed or barguthti while the fairer P. ovata is called isabghol or horse flower.

Growing psyllium

Psyllium is a common herb in India. It can grow to about a foot and half. The leaves are slender and the numerous but small, white flowers grow out of the base of the plant. The flower spikes will change to reddish brown when ripe and the lower leaves will dry out. Its seeds are often found in capsules which open by themselves when ripe. The tap root is well-developed with some fibrous secondary roots.

Psyllium grows well in cool, dry weather which is often sown after the rainy season. It needs a moderate amount of water and will flourish in clear, sunny and dry weather. The soil must be light, sandy loams which do not need to be fertilised. Fields are often irrigated before seeds are sown. Mature psyllium is harvested by cutting at least six inches above ground and bound for drying. It is eventually thrashed and winnowed before the harvested seeds are collected. It is then dried before being cleaned, milled, and stored.

Benefits of psyllium

Psyllium is a popular ingredient in laxatives and in cereals for its soluble fibre. It has benefited people who suffer from constipation, those who do not consume enough roughage, and people who should not be straining their bowel movements. It has also been prescribed for people who suffer from watery diarrhoea. Some people have taken psyllium to aid in lowering their cholesterol levels or to stabilise their blood sugar levels. Psyllium is classified as a bulk laxative. It can absorb water from the intestines and increase stool bulk, making it easy to pass.

What to look out for

Although generally safe, psyllium is not to be taken by people with specific medical conditions. People with blocked intestines, appendicitis, have difficulty swallowing, experienced a sudden change in bowel movements that has lasted longer than two weeks, and rectal bleeding should inform their healthcare provider first before taking anything that has psyllium.

Do not take psyllium for anything longer than seven days without the approval of your physician. Drink every capsule with a full glass of water so it gets flushed out of the throat and down to your stomach. Failure to do so might cause psyllium to swell in the throat and cause choking. Some products might contain sugar or aspartame to improve psyllium's tastelessness. Diabetics, phenylketonurics and conditions that require limiting these substances should ask the pharmacist or chemist about using alternatives.

Possible side effects to watch out for when taking psyllium are flatulence and bloating. Drinking plenty of water will offer some relief. Other less common side effects that people have related to psyllium are cramps, nausea and vomiting, difficulty breathing or swallowing, and skin rash. Other people are sensitive to psyllium, especially when they inhale the fibres.

Psyllium can interact with some medication because it affects the latter's absorption. Tricyclic antidepressants such as amitriptyline, imipramine, and doxepin as well as seizure medications such as carbamazepine should be used with caution. Cholesterol lowering medicines that sequester bile acids and maintenance medications for diabetes and heart disease can also be affected. If possible, take psyllium two to four hours before or after taking any of these medications.

How to use psyllium

Psyllium may be sold as dried seeds or as husks. Commercial preparations appear as wither powder, capsule, tablet or wafer. The seeds can be chewed to extract the almost tasteless mucilage. Its onset of action is about 12 to 24 hours but the full effect may take about two to three days.

Dosages on products that contain psyllium are highly dependent on the labelled instruction. In general, adults can take three to six grams of psyllium powder mixed in eight ounces of water twice or thrice daily. Another full glass of water may be taken after to prevent constipation. Children aged six years and older can consume about 1.5 to three grams dissolved in about four to eight ounces of water every two to three times daily.

Studies on psyllium

Although popular for their husks' fibre content, psyllium seeds contain a mix of polysaccharides such as pentoses, hexoses, and uronic acids. The seed contains about 47 per cent soluble fibre by weight while the husks are made of 67 to 71 per cent soluble fibre, about 85 per cent of total fibre by weight. It is resistant to fermentation as 24 per cent of its arabinose and 53 per cent of its xylose sugars are digestible.

Most of the studies about psyllium focused on its effectiveness for constipation. Consuming 10 grams daily or about 3.6 grams of psyllium thrice daily for two weeks have produced favourable results compared to placebo. A separate study studied the effects of celandine, aloe, and psyllium compared to psyllium. According to their data, those who were able to take the herbs were able to have regular bowel movements and softer stools compared to placebo.

@Arthur Bramble@

Conflicting results have come up from researchers who wanted to see if psyllium is any good in keeping bad cholesterol in check. There is a study that showed psyllium does not significantly lower the cholesterol levels of the participants who have normal or slightly higher cholesterol levels. Separate reviews have demonstrated data in favour of psyllium that it can reduce total cholesterol and bad cholesterol, especially in subjects that have mild to moderately elevated cholesterols even on a low fat diet. A small study has shown psyllium benefiting postmenopausal women in lowering their cholesterol levels and in turn, reduces the incidence of heart disease.

Other smaller studies have been able to demonstrate that psyllium can benefit people with hypertension and maintain normal glucose levels in people affected with type II diabetes.

References:

• A Modern Herbal. "A Modern Herbal | Plantain, Psyllium." 2004. http://botanical.com/botanical/mgmh/p/plapsy47.html (accessed 18 Jun 2013).

• Healthline. "What is Psyllium? Dosing, Side Effects & More." 2005. http://www.healthline.com/natstandardcontent/psyllium (accessed 18 Jun 2013).

• Medline Plus. "Psyllium: MedlinePlus Drug Information." 2010. http://www.nlm.nih.gov/medlineplus/druginfo/meds/a601104.html (accessed 18 Jun 2013).

•   Medscape. "Medscape: Psyllium." 2013.
http://reference.medscape.com/drug/fiberall-metamucil-psyllium-342028 (accessed 18 Jun 2013).

University of Maryland Medical Center. "Psyllium." 2010.
http://umm.edu/health/medical/altmed/supplement/psyllium
(accessed 18 Jun 2013).

HERBAL REMEDIES Q-Z

ROSEMARY- Rosemary is a fragrant shrub native to the Mediterranean and has been valued as a spice, fragrance, and as an herbal remedy for improving memory. Its scientific name is Rosmarinus officinalis. The name comes from the Latin terms "ros" and "marinus" meaning dew of the sea, as the plant subsists on nothing more than the humidity provided by distant sea breeze. It has also been called the compass plant and old man.

Growing rosemary

Rosemary is a small evergreen plant that has leaves that are similar to hemlock's needle like leaves. It may appear upright or trailing to about five feet tall. The leaves are long, narrow and are silver white underneath with dense, woolly hairs. The flowers can range from white, pink, purple, or blue which bloom in spring and summer of temperate climates and year round in warmer regions.

From May through July, rosemary is at its peak and usually harvested. The upper parts of the shoots are stripped off. The oil of rosemary is distilled from the flower's calices but it can be extracted from the stems and leaves.

Rosemary is a hardy plant that can withstand droughts for long periods of time. It is easy to grow and pest resistant. It flourishes in sandy loam soil with good drainage under the full sun. It is often propagated through clippings of the shoot and planting it directly into the soil.

Rosemary can be propagated with seeds, cuttings, and root division. Seeds are often sown under the full sun. Cuttings are often taken in August, about half a foot long and planted two-thirds in the ground. Once rooted, it can be transplanted to its permanent location. The herb prefers light, dry soil with a light shade. Most herbalists prefer plants grown from seeds.

Benefits of rosemary

Fragrant rosemary is often associated for the flavours and aroma it has always imparted to rich food. It has components that can stimulate the immune system, enhance blood circulation, and improve digestion. It has been utilised for asthma and any form of inflammation in the body. It's a traditional herbal remedy for renal colic and painful menstruation. The herbal extracts have been found effective for hair loss, although in combination with other herbs. Other cultures have prescribed rosemary for diabetes and high blood pressure. Aroma therapists have banked on its fragrance in relieving anxiety and stress while cosmetologists have long relied on the herb for removing cellulite and wrinkles.

What to look out for

When eaten in amounts found in food, rosemary is generally safe. It is usually safe in amounts used as medicine. However, the oil must be diluted before use. Consuming large amounts of rosemary will cause vomiting, bleeding in the uterus, irritation of the kidneys, increased sensitivity of the skin to sunlight, and allergic reactions. It has also been reported that volatile oil from rosemary can be irritating to the mucous membranes lining the intestines which can cause nausea and cramping.

Pregnant and breastfeeding women as well as people with seizure and bone problems should not use rosemary as herbal remedy. Rosemary oil can cause contact dermatitis, occupational asthma, and inflamed lips. Rosemary can trigger oestrogen deficiencies, increase in blood sugar, and low blood pressure. Despite rosemary not being a diuretic, it can increase excretion of electrolytes such as sodium, potassium, and chloride which can decrease creatinine clearance.

How to use rosemary

The leaves of the rosemary have been used for culinary dishes and herbal medicine. When eaten, it has a strong lemon-pine flavour and a spicy pine aroma. Germany's Commission E has approved the use of rosemary leaves for dyspepsia and the external use of the oil for joint pains and inadequate blood circulation in the limbs.

Commercially, rosemary is available as a dried whole herb, encapsulated as a dried, powdered extract, and as a volatile oil. Traditional preparations of rosemary are also available as teas, alcohol tinctures, and liquid extracts. Total daily intake of the herb should not exceed four to six grams of the dried herb.

The essential oil of rosemary has been combined with thyme, cedar wood, lavender, jojoba, and grape seed oil for bald spots. The mixture is massaged on the scalp for about a minute or two with a warm towel placed around it to increase absorption. As a tea, a gram or two of the dried herb or young tops, leaves and flowers is steeped in 150 millilitres of water for 10 minutes to make a cup. It can be taken every eight hours for dyspepsia, hypertension, or rheumatism. Alternatively, a dose of two to four millilitres of rosemary extract is given thrice daily. It can also be made into a preserve by mixing one part of fresh rosemary tops with three parts of sugar. Fresh sprigs of rosemary can be mixed in wine to relieve heart palpitations, headache relief, and act as a mild diuretic. Rosemary and coltsfoot leaves may be rubbed and smoked for asthma and other lung and throat disorders.

Studies on rosemary

Rosemary contains caffeic acid and rosmarinic acid as its active components. These compounds are powerful antioxidants and have been researched for their potential in curing some cancers, liver problems, and inflammatory conditions. Its volatile oil contains borneol, camphor, cineol, pinene, and camphene. It appears colourless with a warm camphor-like taste. A 100 pound flowering rosemary tops will yield eight ounces of the oil.

There is a poorly designed study which demonstrated that rosemary along with other herbs can be used for falling hair. The study involved 84 participants suffering from bald spots and has massaged their scalp daily for seven months. The essential oils have significant hair growth compared to the placebo. Several studies focused on rosemary's effect on food preservation. According to most of their data, rosemary has been able to inhibit foodborne pathogens such as Listeria monocytogenes, Bacillus cereus, and Staphylococcus aureus. A separate study has suggested that rosemary oil, when used in aroma therapy, has been able to lower cortisol levels and anxiety.

References:

•   Discovery Fit and Health. "Discovery Health "Herbs: Rosemary Fact Sheet"." 2010. http://health.howstuffworks.com/wellness/food-nutrition/natural-foods/herbs-rosemary-fact-sheet.htm (accessed 19 Jun 2013).

•   Healthline. "What is Rosemary? Dosing, Side Effects & More." 2006. http://www.healthline.com/natstandardcontent/rosemary (accessed 19 Jun 2013).

•   RxList. "Rosemary Effectiveness, Safety, and Drug Interactions on RxList." 2013.

http://www.rxlist.com/rosemary/supplements.htm (accessed 19 Jun 2013).

• University of Maryland Medical Center. "Rosemary." 2004. http://umm.edu/health/medical/altmed/herb/rosemary (accessed 19 Jun 2013).

World's Healthiest Foods. "Rosemary." 2009. http://www.whfoods.com/genpage.php?tname=foodspice&dbid=7 5 (accessed 19 Jun 2013).

SAGE- Sage is a small, perennial, evergreen shrub used for cooking and herbal medicine. Its scientific name is Salvia officinalis although most people call it common sage, broadleaf sage or garden sage. It's also called in other languages as adacayi, maramia, and sauge. It is a local plant in the Mediterranean but has been cultivated in other places. The term "sage" can also refer to other plants. The term "salvia" comes from the Latin salvere, meaning to save. It refers to the herb's healing properties.

Growing sage

Although referred to as an herb, sage is a small shrub. It has woody stems, greyish green leaves, and has blue to purplish flowers. It can grow up to two feet tall and will often bloom in late spring or summer. The leaves are oval and will range in size, depending on the cultivar, but will be creased on top and will appear white underneath because of the numerous short fuzzy hairs. It is often arranged in pairs and oval in shape with rounded ends. The flowers are arranged in whorls and often bloom in August. The whole plant will have a strong scent and somewhat warm and bitter due to its volatile oils.

Sage has been cultivated for centuries as food and medicine. It can be grown from seeds or through summer cuttings. It prefers a warm but dry plot, although slightly shaded on ordinary garden soil. It is a hardy plant but will not last three to four years before degenerating. This is why new sage seedlings are planted every four years. Cuttings may also be taken in autumn, after the plants have stopped flowering.

Benefits of sage

Ancient herbalists have written about a variety of uses for the plant. It has been grown in some parts of Europe for its essential oil. Many European dishes have sage as and ingredient, except for French cuisine. It offers a wide variety of medicinal benefits, especially in traditional remedies. Modern science suggests that sage has antiperspirant, antimicrobial, astringent, antispasmodic, hypoglycemic, oestrogenic, and tonic effects.

What to look out for

As it is widely used as a spice, sage is relatively safe. However, there is limited information on sage's safety. However, sage essential oil contains thujone, a known neurotoxin which can cause seizures in large amounts. It can also damage the liver and the nervous system. Maximum safety dose have not been determined. Ingesting 12 drops or more of the essential oil is lethal. It is also a potent uterine stimulant so pregnant women should steer clear of this herb, including nursing women. People with seizure disorders or diabetic should also not use sage.

People using sage as an herbal remedy have reported experiencing nausea and vomiting, stomach pain, light-headedness, tension, and breathlessness. Headaches and irritability have also been observed in people who consume too much sage in their diet.

Some medications can interact with the use of sage. With anti-diabetes medication such as glyburide, insulin, rosiglitazone, chlorpropamide and the like, sage might lower blood sugar too much. Sage can also decrease the effectiveness of anticonvulsants such as barbiturates, valproic acid, gabapentin, phenytoin, and other similar medications. Sedatives such as lorazepam, zolpidem and the like mixed in with sage might depress the central nervous system too much.

How to use sage

Mediterranean folk remedies use sage for heavy, menstrual bleeding, improve fertility, enhance memory, relieve symptoms of arthritis, and ease breast engorgement during weaning. It has been applied locally for wounds, sprains, and muscle injuries. Sage extracts can be gargled for sore throat, hoarseness, and dry cough.

Germany's Commission E has approved the internal use of sage for dyspepsia and excessive sweating along with its topical application for inflamed nasal passages and throat. It has been listed in the

United States Pharmacopoeia from 1840 to 1900. At present, sage is listed under the generally recognised as safe (GRAS) category.

Fresh sage leaves are rubbed on teeth to clean them and to strengthen the gums. Herbal based dental powders will often contain sage. It can also be rubbed on skin abrasions or used as poultice for ulcers and wounds.

If used as tea or gargle, one to three grams of dried sage is steeped in a cup of boiling water for 10 to 15 minutes and taken thrice daily. It can be inhaled for asthma attacks or to remove mucus congestion in the airways. For improved memory and concentration, a dose of 300 to 600 milligrams of dried sage leaf has been found effective. Alcoholic sage extracts have been given at 333 milligrams or up to 1000 milligrams by mouth daily.

It has been mixed in a cream with rhubarb and applied on cold sores. The cream is made up of 23 grams of sage and rhubarb extract has been applied every two to four hours on cold sores from the first day the symptoms appear up to two weeks. It can be used as a hair rinse for dandruff and to restore color to greying hair.

Studies on sage

The most potent substances of sage are found in its essential oil. It contains cineole, borneol, and thujone. The leaves are abundant with tannic, oleic, ursonic, ursolic, cornsolic, fumaric, chlorogenic, and caffeic acids aside from niacin, nicotinamide, flavones, and flavonoid glycosides. It will appear yellow or greenish-yellow with penetrating odour.

Many scientific investigations have zeroed in on sage as a potential treatment for Alzheimer's disease. A double blind, randomised, placebo controlled trial has suggested that sage can manage mild to moderate cases of Alzheimer's disease. Separate studies investigated whether sage can improve mental function and mood swings. Although most are poorly designed and involved a small number of participants, their data has been able to suggest that sage can improve some mental faculties plus it can improve mood and anxiety levels.

Sage leaf extract may be an effective and safe alternative in hyperlipedimia. The small randomised trial was able to demonstrate that using 500 milligrams every eight hours can lower total cholesterol and bad cholesterol levels.

References:

- Discovery Fit and Health. "Discovery Health "Sage: Herbal Remedies"." 2013. http://health.howstuffworks.com/wellness/natural-medicine/herbal-remedies/sage-herbal-remedies.htm (accessed 19 Jun 2013).

- Health from Nature. "Sage - Salvia officinalis | Medicinal use, description and other useful informations about Sage." 2011. http://health-from-nature.net/Sage.html (accessed 19 Jun 2013).

- Herb Wisdom. "Sage Benefits & Information." 2005. http://www.herbwisdom.com/herb-sage.html (accessed 19 Jun 2013).

- RxList. "Sage Effectiveness, Safety, and Drug Interactions on RxList." 2013. http://www.rxlist.com/sage/supplements.htm (accessed 19 Jun 2013).

- Willis-Knighton Health System. "Sage - Health Library - Willis-Knighton Health System - Shreveport - Bossier City, Louisiana." 2012. http://healthlibrary.wkhs.com/article.aspx?chunkiid=1118 02 (accessed 19 Jun 2013).

SAW PALMETTO- Saw palmetto is a slightly small palm tree that has berry-like fruits that have been popularly used for the treatment of enlarged prostate. Its scientific name is Serenoa repens and is also known by other names as American dwarf palm tree, palmetto scrub, and cabbage palm.

Growing saw palmetto

A native of south eastern United States, saw palmetto is often found along the Atlantic and Gulf coast, but it can grow inland down to southern Arkansas. This is a resilient plant that grows slowly but lives for a long time. Native Americans have used the berries for men with urinary conditions and for women with breast disorders. The Mayans have used it as a tonic while the Seminoles employed the berries as an herbal expectorant and antiseptic.

Saw palmetto is a rather small fan palm. It grows from three to six feet with the trunk spread out and growing in tufts. The leaves are smooth and shiny, with its bare petiole ending in a wide fan with about 20 leaflets. Leaves are about three to seven feet long, its leaflets at 20 to 39 inches long. The yellowish white flowers form a thick clump of small flowerets of about 24 inches long. The large, edible drupe is bitter when green and unripe but becomes palatable when it turns reddish-black.

Benefits of saw palmetto

The fruits of the saw palmetto have been under scrutiny for its fatty acids and phytosterols that have shown potential for benign prostatic enlargement (BPH). The extracts have also been given for baldness, polycystic ovarian syndrome (PCOS) and other conditions caused by an overabundance of androgenic hormones in the body. Aside from enlarged prostate, it has also treated sore testicles and inflammation of the urinary tract. Saw palmetto has also been employed for relieving mucus congestion in the respiratory tract, fortify the thyroid, and stabilise the body's metabolism. It has also been utilised for improving appetite and digestion, improve breast size and appearance, and improve sexual performance.

What to look out for

People who have used saw palmetto extract might experience mild stomach upset, nausea, irregular bowel movements, dry mouth, bad breath, liver irritation, and peptic ulcer. Some people have also reported mild headache, light-headedness, insomnia, and depression. It can also cause difficulty getting an erection and dwindling sex drive in males.

Certain conditions should not be using saw palmetto as it might get worse. People with bleeding disorders, gastrointestinal problems, and hormone affective conditions should consult their health provider first before using this supplement. It might also aggravate people with hypertension. Its effect on hormones meant that pregnant and lactating women should never use this.

There is a rare incidence of bleeding while on saw palmetto so people with scheduled surgery or any medical or dental procedure should stop using this supplement at least two weeks before the set date. Those taking saw palmetto tinctures should not engage in activities that require concentration and focus as it contains high amounts of alcohol.

Some herbs and dietary supplements might interact with saw palmetto. Red clover and soy beans have oestrogen-like properties which can interfere with the effects of saw palmetto. Certain preparations containing saw palmetto might increase the risk of bleeding when used with ginkgo and garlic. It might interact with medications that affect blood coagulation as well as drugs that contain sex hormones.

How to use saw palmetto

Like most supplements, using saw palmetto is dependent on the labelled instructions of the manufacturer. There is no standard dose for saw palmetto, as the doses are often based on scientific studies and traditional use. It is recommended that you consult your health provider first before using it.

Traditionally, berried have been taken for saw palmetto's full effect. A dose of one or two grams of dried, ground or whole berries have been consumed daily. Teas are often made from berries but researchers are doubtful if it has any effect as it does not dissolve in water. If saw palmetto tincture is used, a dose of two to four millilitres are given every eight hours in a day. The fluid extract of the berry pulp may be given at one to two millilitres taken thrice daily. An experimental dosage form of saw palmetto is in a 640 milligram rectal suppository that is given once daily, although it has not been proven to be more effective than when taking saw palmetto by mouth. People suffering from benign prostatic hyperplasia take 160 milligrams of saw palmetto every 12 hours.

Saw palmetto oil is a recognised treatment for benign prostatic hyperplasia in New Zealand, France, Germany and many European countries. It has been listed in the United States Pharmacopoeia from 1906 to 1917 and in the National Formulary from 1926 to 1950.

Studies on saw palmetto

The exact mechanism of action why saw palmetto works is not yet known but researchers have numerous hypotheses. Saw palmetto is believed to inhibit an enzyme, 5-alpha-reductase, which explains its anti-testosterone activities. However, it does not explain why saw palmetto has anti-inflammatory properties and its other hormonal effects.

Clinical trials have been done on the extracts of saw palmetto and its apparent effect compared to other drugs, such as finasteride and tamsulosin, on people with mild to moderate BPH. However, larger studies have shown that saw palmetto's effect is no different from the placebo. Anecdotal evidence from people with hyperplasia has been able to show that saw palmetto extract can reduce their problems in the bladder.

Problems in the male urinary tract and whether saw palmetto extract is helpful have been studied and the results are conflicting. A single study has suggested that saw palmetto extract can reduce the incidence of hair loss, especially those caused by hormonal imbalance. Some athletes have used saw palmetto as a steroid substitute to increase muscle mass. Herbalists agree that saw palmetto can prevent muscle wasting and have used it for emaciating diseases. Nevertheless, more studies should be done in order to show saw palmetto's effectiveness for these conditions.

References:

• Medline Plus. "Saw palmetto: MedlinePlus Supplements." 2012. http://www.nlm.nih.gov/medlineplus/druginfo/natural/971.html (accessed 20 Jun 2013).

• Mayo Clinic. "Saw palmetto (Serenoa repens [Bartram] Small) - MayoClinic.com." 2012. http://www.mayoclinic.com/health/saw-palmetto/NS_patient-sawpalmetto (accessed 20 Jun 2013).

• Intelihealth. "Saw Palmetto - Index of Herbal Medicines, Supplements and Therapies - Complementary & Alternative Medicine | Aetna InteliHealth." 2008. http://www.intelihealth.com/IH/ihtIH/E/8513/31402/346487.html?d=dmtContent (accessed 20 Jun 2013).

• Herb Wisdom. "Saw palmetto Benefits & Information." 2009. http://www.herbwisdom.com/herb-saw-palmetto.html (accessed 20 Jun 2013).

• Health Library by iHerb. "Health Library - C573 - Saw Palmetto - Natural, Alternative - 21865." 2010. http://healthlibrary.epnet.com/GetContent.aspx?token=e0498803-7f62-4563-8d47-5fe33da65dd4&chunkiid=21865 (accessed 20 Jun 2013).

SCULLCAP – Skullcap is a member of the mint family that has a diverse use in herbal medicine. The most popular in North American medicine is Scutellaria laterifolia or the Virginian skullcap. It has also been called blue pimpernel, hoodwort, mad dog weed, helmet flower, and Quaker bonnet. The term skullcap refers to the plant's helmet-like calyx on the outer spiral of small flowers.

Growing skullcap

The American skullcap grows upright at about two to three feet in height. It has spear-like leaves. The blue or purplish-blue flowers appear at the side branches that come from the leaf axils. Flowers often bloom in July. The whole herb is often harvested by June. It is then dried and powdered. The skullcap has different varieties and is found abundantly in Europe and Asia. American skullcap is native to large regions of North America.

Skullcap flourishes best in wetlands. It is found often in marshes and meadows. The seeds of the skullcap can be sown during temperate February or March outdoors where it can be lightly shaded. Root divisions can be transplanted in March or April. Whether from seed or root division, the skullcap can be transferred to its permanent plot by autumn. It can grow in ordinary garden soil, although it prefers sunny, open plots of land. These herbs live for about two to three to four years.

Benefits of skullcap

Skullcap is a popular herbal sedative and sleep inducer. It has also been given to manage stroke, seizures, ticks, and anxiety. Another alternative benefit skullcap might provide is its ability to lower blood pressure, ease out menstrual cramps, and as an aid for alcohol and tobacco. Skullcap is a trusted home remedy for hiccups, hangovers, and asthma. Traditionally, skullcap has been prescribed in the 18th century for rabies, hence the name mad dog weed. It may also be given for joint pains, attention deficit-hyperactive disorder (ADHD), and for increase muscle bulk. This herb is popular in Northern America but very few people outside the region use it.

What to look out for

There is very little data about the safety of skullcap. There are reports from the Netherlands and Norway on people using skullcap developed liver problems. However, advocates of the herb believe it is due to adulteration with germander. In the United States, there are no reports on any adverse effects caused by skullcap consumption. Large amounts of skullcap tincture can cause light-headedness, convulsions, erratic pulse, and tremors. Skullcap has also been given for high cholesterol, fever, hardening of the arteries, skin infections, and skin allergies.

Until more data is known, pregnant and breastfeeding women should not use it. Initial investigation has shown skullcap can prevent sex and pituitary hormones. People using skullcap should avoid driving or operating heavy machinery as it causes drowsiness. For this reason, discontinue skullcap use two weeks before any scheduled medical procedure such as surgeries because it might interact with anaesthetics and blood pressure medications. Other common side effects in using skullcap include diarrhoea and stomach upset. When gastrointestinal side effects appear, either the dose is reduced or you should stop using it.

Skullcap can be used in combination with oats and St. John's wort safely. It also works well in combination with other sedative herbs such as valerian, passionflower, and black cohosh. However, skullcap can interact with other sedating medications such as antihistamines, barbiturates, and benzodiazepines.

How to use skullcap

Skullcap is often sold commercially as a tea, liquid extract, dried powder, and in capsules. If used fresh, the leaves and stems of the American skullcap is used.

Skullcap tea is made by steeping a teaspoon or two of 250 millilitres boiling water for 10 to 15 minutes to make one cup. About two to three cups may be taken daily. For those who prefer the liquid tincture, two to four millilitres of the skullcap solution is mixed in 250 millilitres of warm water and can be taken every eight hours. Homemade skullcap tincture can be made by steeping one part of fresh herb in five parts water or alcohol.

The dried herb can also be sewn into eight square inches of cloth as an herbal pillow for insomnia. This herbal pillow is placed under the usual bed pillow to ease insomnia. About 195 milligrams of the dried skullcap powder has been given to relieve hiccups.

Studies on skullcap

Skullcap is rich in flavonoids such as scutellarin, wogonin, and baicalin which have been identified as the components that exert sedative and anti-spasmodic effects. It is believed that these substances act similar to the body's natural gamma amino butyric acid (GABA). It also contains scutellarein, lateriflorin, biacalein, sugars, and cellulose. Its chrysin content might be helpful for bodybuilders who want to get bigger and stronger muscles.

A double-blind, placebo controlled study has been done to assess the calming effects of skullcap in humans. A small population of volunteers have been able to prove that skullcap has indeed a positive anxiolytic effect in lower doses and an obvious sedating action in higher doses.

@Arthur Bramble@

The teas made from skullcaps in general have been able to show some antibacterial and antifungal effects. However, clinical studies have yet to be done to identify which type of pathogen it can control and whether it has any effect on humans in general in terms of its antimicrobial action.

A research conducted on 55 herbs to assess claims of their antioxidant properties. Skullcap is one of the top five herbs with the highest ability to rein in on free radicals, higher than milk thistle and tea leaf. This is the basis of some herbalists that use skullcap for kidney conditions.

In 2012, a study in mice infected with prions is treated with skullcap. According to their data, the extracts from skullcap have been able to delay its onset. The active components used are flavonoids baicalein and baicalin which are given orally. These properties have spurred more research focused on developing medicines for prion diseases and neurodegenerative conditions such as Alzheimer's and Parkinson's disease.

References:

• A Modern Herbal. "A Modern Herbal | Scullcaps." 2008. http://botanical.com/botanical/mgmh/s/scullc34.html#vir (accessed 20 Jun 2013).

• Discovery Fit and Health. "Discovery Health "Skullcap: Herbal Remedies"." 2007.

http://health.howstuffworks.com/wellness/natural-medicine/herbal-remedies/skullcap-herbal-remedies.htm (accessed 20 Jun 2013).

• Drugs.com. "Scullcap professional information from Drugs.com." 2003. http://www.drugs.com/npp/scullcap.html (accessed 20 Jun 2013).

• University of Maryland Medical Center. "Skullcap." 2003. http://umm.edu/health/medical/altmed/herb/skullcap (accessed 20 Jun 2013).

WebMD. "SKULLCAP: Uses, Side Effects, Interactions and Warnings - WebMD." 2009. http://www.webmd.com/vitamins-supplements/ingredientmono-986-SKULLCAP.aspx?activeIngredientId=986&activeIngredientName=S KULLCAP (accessed 20 Jun 2013).

SHEPHERD'S PURSE- Shepherd's purse is a weed known for its triangular seed pods that look like a purse. It's related to the mustard and is known for its scientific name Capsella bursa-pastoris. It has also been called blind weed, cocowort, mother's heart, pepper-and-salt, rattle pouches, shovel weed, and toywort.

Growing shepherd's purse

Although shepherd's purse is native to eastern parts of Europe and some parts of Asia Minor, it has became a common weed in most parts of the world, especially those in colder climates. It is often found in disturbed areas, along roadsides and gardens.

Shepherd's purse grows from the rosette of round toothed leaves at its base. A stem often comes out from it. It has small white flowers that look like dandelions which blooms all year long. However, it does not have milky-white sap and its lobed leaves point outward. The flowers have four petals and often appear in round clusters before it becomes elongated and become fruit or more technically, a seed pod. This ability to have hardy flowers makes them capable of reproducing several generations annual through its seeds. The yellow, oblong seeds are enclosed in seed pods that are heart shaped and flat. Seeds are often numerous and have miniscule, netlike patterns. It also has a slender, white taproot.

Benefits of shepherd's purse

Medicinally, shepherd's purse is just as valuable for its ability to stop bleeding by constricting blood vessels. It has been given for disinfecting the liver and the urinary tract as well as easing out bouts of diarrhoea. It is a natural remedy for menstrual cramps as well as managing muscle problems and circulatory disorders. It relieves stress and has been employed in traditional Chinese medicine as an eye tonic and as a contraceptive.

Shepherd's purse is an edible plant. Its flowers, leaves, and seeds have been used as pot herb. The young leaves can be eaten raw or cooked. It is rich in choline, thiamine, inositol, and fumaric acid. It also has riboflavin, ascorbic acid, and minerals such as calcium, phosphorus, and potassium. Traces of vitamin K, beta carotene, iron, niacin, and rutin have also been found in trace amounts.

What to look out for

Shepherd's purse can cause some side effects. It can cause sleepiness, drastic lowering of blood pressure, changes in thyroid function, and heart palpitations. As such, people with scheduled surgery or medical procedures should stop using it at least two weeks before the appointment because it might cause extreme drowsiness. Rarely, it might trigger an allergy which might cause shortness of breath. An overdose of shepherd's purse can cause muscle paralysis, breathing problems, and death.

Although very useful, shepherd's purse should never be used in high doses for a prolonged period of time. Pregnant women should not use shepherd's purse because it might cause uterine contractions. This has been ranked 7th of the 250 anti-fertility plants in China. People with heart problems, kidney stones, and thyroid conditions should avoid shepherd's purse without the supervision of your health provider.

Shepherd's purse should be used with caution with people taking sedatives and thyroid hormones. High doses of the herb can cause too much sleepiness when used with sedative medications such as clonazepam, phenobarbital, zolpidem and the like. Sodium oxybate, a prescription medicine given for narcoleptics, and shepherd's purse might cancel each other's effects. Shepherd's purse can also inhibit thyroid hormones so this might decrease the potency of thyroid medications.

Dried shepherd's purse does not keep their potency longer than a year. Fresh herbs are more potent or its tinctures retain its medicinal activity.

How to use shepherd's purse

Like the dandelion, shepherd's purse is highly edible when young. It has been gathered in the wild or even cultivated for food. Shanghai stir fries this in rice cakes or as a wonton filling. South Koreans cook it in a vegetable side dish. It tastes like mild radish. Its peppery seeds have been used as mild spice for salad greens.

Bleeding can be stopped by putting 10 millilitres of shepherd's purse every 15 minutes while applying direct pressure. Alternatively, a poultice of the herb may also do. If that's too messy, drinking two cups of cold tea every hour will have the same effect. The tea is also used as an herbal diuretic, hypotensive, vasoconstrictor, and anti-scurvy. The juice of the herb may be placed on cotton wool and applied for nose bleeds.

There are no standard doses for shepherd's purse. However, there are doses that have been used in research and tradition that have been found to exert some medicinal effects. When taken orally, one to four grams of the herb can be taken by mouth every eight hours daily. When crushed, a dose of 10 to 15 grams per day may be divided into three equally divided doses. Liquid extracts containing shepherd's purse may be given at about five to eight grams daily and divided into two to three doses. If applied topically, about three to five grams of the herb will do.

The tincture of shepherd's purse can be made by filling a bottle with 1/3 of loose dried herbs or ¾ parts with fresh herbs before filling it with vodka. Screw the lid on and leave it to set for six to eight weeks. Before using, it should be strained well. An infusion of the herb may be done by boiling 250 millilitres of water to an ounce of the herb for about 10 to 15 minutes and then strained before being drank cold.

Studies on shepherd's purse

Fumaric acid is one of the active principles found in shepherd's purse. Fumaric acid is an anti-cancer substance that has demonstrated to limit certain types of cancer strains in mice. Its active constituent has been called bursinic acid and it also has an alkaloid, bursine, which resembles sulphocyansinapine in structure. It also contains sulphurated oil, similar to mustard oil that gives off its pungent, cress-like odour. Its rich oxalate content has made it hazardous for people with kidney stones to take.

References:

• A Modern Herbal. "A Modern Herbal | Shepherd's Purse." n.d.. http://botanical.com/botanical/mgmh/s/shephe47.html (accessed 21 Jun 2013).

• Discovery Fit and Health. "Discovery Health "Shepherd's Purse: Herbal Remedies"." 2010. http://health.howstuffworks.com/wellness/natural-medicine/herbal-remedies/shepherds-purse-herbal-remedies.htm (accessed 21 Jun 2013).

• Medscape. "Medscape: Shepherd's purse." 2013. http://reference.medscape.com/drug/blindweed-caseweed-shephards-purse-344454 (accessed 21 Jun 2013).

• RxList. "Shepherd's Purse Effectiveness, Safety, and Drug Interactions on RxList." 2013. http://www.rxlist.com/shepherds_purse/supplements.htm (accessed 21 Jun 2013).

WebMD. "SHEPHERD'S PURSE: Uses, Side Effects, Interactions and Warnings - WebMD." 2009. http://www.webmd.com/vitamins-supplements/ingredientmono-51-SHEPHERD'S%20PURSE.aspx?activeIngredientId=51&activeIngredientName=SHEPHERD'S%20PURSE (accessed 21 Jun 2013).

SLIPPERY ELM- In the past it was primarily used on skin injuries like chapped lips and burns as a salve. Mucilage can be found in the bark of the elm, a gelatin like substance which when placed in water swells. When ingested or applied to wounds this mucilage would coat the area and provide relief.

Nowadays slippery elm is typically used in lozenges to relieve smokers cough and the pain that comes with a sore throat. In a powder form the bark can be used to treat minor wounds, boils and burns.

Slippery elm is a tree that has a mucilaginous inner bark and leaves that are used as herbal remedies. Its scientific name is Ulmus rubra. The Indian, moose, soft, red and sweet elms refer to this tree. The term "rubra" means red, which alludes to the wood that has reddish tint.

Growing slippery elm

Slippery elm is a native tree of North America. The tree grows in moist, shady woodlands, along stream banks, and in any soil that is rich in compost and often moist.

The woody slippery elm can grow up to 65 feet tall with a trunk that can be as wide as 20 inches. The branches are often upright and not numerous compared to the typical American elm. Its crown is made of spreading branches. Its inner wood is reddish-brown in colour. Its yellowish orange-tipped buds and twigs are furry. The rough, dark green leaves are about four to six inches long and will have unevenly toothed margins. The flowers lack petals and often rely on the wind for pollination. Short stalked flowers come in clusters and bloom in the early spring. The fruits are flattened ovals with wings that are about 20 millimetres long. It contains a single seed in its centre.

The inner bark of the slippery elm is harvested in spring or fall. It will appear white to pink and smells like maple syrup when dried. Herbalists recommend using 10 year old bark for herbal remedies. The course powder is for external use while fine, powdered bark is for mucilaginous drink. It should appear grayish or beige and should be checked for starch or damaged flour as adulterants. Moistened bark can be molded into suppositories and lozenges.

Benefits of slippery elm

As an herbal remedy, slippery elm is valued for its mucilage which acts as a demulcent for the skin and the digestive tract as well as antitussive for the respiratory system. Its gruel has been given as nutrient for people recovering from disease including those suffering from diarrhoea and sore throat. It can also be employed as a bulk laxative and for people trying to lose weight. It has been applied on the skin affected with boils, wounds, and burns for its soothing effect. The herb is listed as an official drug of the United States Pharmacopoeia.

Native Americans and early settlers have been using the inner bark of the slippery elm mostly for digestive problems such as diarrhea or constipation. Civil war soldiers have applied it to sustained gunshot wounds to draw out its poison. It's an effective herbal remedy that has been recognized by the United States Food and Drugs Administration (US FDA) as an over-the-counter remedy. It is considered as survival food.

What to look out for

Slippery elm should not be used by people with blocked intestines. The water retaining property of slippery elm might worsen the obstructions. The same is true for people taking slippery elm orally. Every dose should be taken with a generous amount of water to lower the risk of blocking the esophagus. Because of this property, slippery elm can decrease the absorption of some medications. It can be avoided by taking slippery elm an hour or two after taking regular medications.

Children younger than two years old should use slippery elm with caution. Some find it difficult to swallow either tea or gruel and it must be taken with lots of water. Although completely nontoxic and there are no known drug interactions, slippery elm can trigger skin rash on a minority of people with sensitive skin. Anecdotal evidence has shown that slippery elm can cause miscarriage when inserted in the cervix of pregnant women. Although scientific data has to prove it otherwise, consult a healthcare provider before using it.

How to use slippery elm

The most common dosage for slippery elm is to take four to 10 grams of the encapsulated dried powder of the inner bark. Cough and sore throat lozenges are sucked at a dose of 500 milligrams to one gram thrice daily.

The inner bark is grounded and cooked as porridge. It tastes like porridge but packed with antioxidants. When ground and mixed with boiling water, it becomes a paste that can be applied to wounds, burns, boils, ulcers, and other sore surfaces. Low doses of slippery elm are given for diarrhea while higher doses have a laxative effect. The tea is made by boiling loose bark in a cup of water for 10 to 15 minutes and cooled before drinking. The tea can be taken every six to eight hours daily.

Slippery elm simmered with flax seed, thoroughwort, licorice, and water is strained and mixed with vinegar and sugar for bronchitis. A dose of 15 millilitres is given twice or thrice daily. For pleurisy, orange milkweed root, marshmallow root, licorice root, and slippery elm bark is boiled in water. Taken when warm, a dose of 2.5 millilitres is given every 30 minutes. An enema for diarrhoea, dysentery, and other similar conditions can be made with powdered slippery elm bark, powdered bayberry, and skullcap poured in boiling water and steeped for 30 minutes. It is then strained and mixed with tincture of myrrh before being used tepid.

Commercial preparations of slippery elm come in teas and capsules. Sometimes, it is combined with other herbs such as peppermint, ginger or aloe. When combined with sheep sorrel, burdock root, and Turkish rhubarb, slippery elm becomes one of the essential herbs in Essiac recipe for estrogen sensitive cancers. If combined with prickly ash and juniper berries, burdock, and uva ursi, slippery elm is given as kidney remedy in a patented herbal formula made by Rene Caisse.

Studies on slippery elm

Slippery elm's mucilage is rich in polysaccharides. Galactose and rhamnose are the primary sugars found in the mucilage and some starch, cellulose, and lignins. Other active constituents found in slippery elm are calcium oxalate, phytosterols, sesquiterpenes, flavonoids, salicylic, capric, caprylic, and decanoic acids, and vitamin E. Its tannin content gives it an astringent effect.

References:

• Essiac Facts. "Slippery Elm Bark: A Native Medicine - Essiac Facts." 2013. http://essiacfacts.com/slippery-elm-bark-a-native-medicine/ (accessed 21 Jun 2013).

- Herbal Remedy Pro. "Herbal Remedy: Slippery Elm Bark." 2011. http://www.herbalremedypro.com/slipperyelmbark.htm (accessed 21 Jun 2013).

- Mediherb. "The Numerous Healing Properties of Slippery Elm." 2004. http://www.mediherb.com/pdf/6042.pdf (accessed 21 Jun 2013).

- Mother Earth Herbs. "Mother Earth Herbs - Slippery elm." 2000. http://www.motherearthherbs.com/elm.html (accessed 21 Jun 2013).

Natural Therapy Pages. "Natural Therapy: Slippery Elm." 2004. http://www.naturaltherapypages.com.au/article/slippery_elm (accessed 21 Jun 2013).

ST. JOHN'S WORT – St. John's Wort is a perennial herb native to Europe that is a popular herbal remedy for depression. Its scientific name is Hypericum perforatum and is also called chase devil, goatweed, Tipton's weed, or rosin rose. Sprigs of this herb are often placed above religious icons during this day to ward off evil. The oil glands on the leaves appear like windows when held against the light.

Growing St. John's wort

St. John's wort is an herb that grows wild in temperate climates. It can be found in fallow soil, woodlands, shrubberies, waysides, and paddocks. It is found in Britain and all throughout Europe and Asia.

As a wild herb, St John's wort can grow up to three feet in height. It has short, barren sprouts and upright, smooth stems that branch out on top. Its leaves are pale green, oblong in shape, and have no stalks. Its transparent oil glands are often visible when holding the leaf up to the light. Bright yellow, five petal flowers have marked dots and lines. These flowers blooms June to August. It eventually develops several small and round black seeds contained in a capsule and exudes a resinous aroma.

Benefits of St. John's wort

St John's wort is popular for being an herbal antidepressant. However, the herb has also been given for related conditions migraine headaches, nerve pain, sciatica, and obsessive compulsive behaviour including stomach upset and premenstrual syndrome (PMS). When applied topically, St John's wort is beneficial for muscle pain, minor burns, cuts, and bruises.

What to look out for

When taken short term, St John's wort is safe for most people. However, it can bring about side effects such as insomnia, restlessness, anxiety, irritability, fatigue, dry mouth, light headedness, headache, diarrhoea, and tingling in the extremities. It can also make the skin more sensitive to the ultraviolet rays of the sun which can trigger skin rashes unless you apply sunblock with high sun protection factor (SPF). In published studies, the herb has been well tolerated at recommended dose for up to three months.

Certain conditions should reconsider using St John's wort. Pregnant women and those trying to get pregnant including those who are currently breastfeeding should not use this herb. People with diagnosed attention deficit-hyperactivity disorder (ADHD), bipolar disorder, Alzheimer's diseases, and severe depression must talk to their healthcare provider before using the herb. Those scheduled for surgery or any medical and dental procedure that will require the use of anaesthetics should not use this herb because it might depress the nervous system too much. There are reports of suicidal or homicidal thoughts in some users.

Many medications might interact with St John's wort. When combined with tramadol, sertraline, pentazocine, paroxetine, nefazodone, meperidine, or fenfluramine can cause too much serotonin in the brain which will cause confusion, muscle stiffness, and shivering. Tacrolimus, reserpine, amitriptyline, phenytoin, morphine, alprazolam, imatinib, saquinavir or oral contraceptives can be quickly broken down by the body and make it ineffective when used with this herb. Phenobarbital can cause extreme sedation when taken with St John's wort. Photosensitising medications such as ciprofloxacin, co-trimoxazole, tetracycline, or methoxypsoralen will increase the risk of sunburn when used with St John's wort. Digoxin's absorption by the body is affected by St John's wort and renders it ineffective.

How to use St. John's wort

For mild to moderate depression, standardised extract of St John's wort containing 0.3 per cent hypericin can be taken at 300 milligrams every eight hours. Children can also take this extract but at a dose of 300 milligrams daily. For standardised extracts that contain 0.2 per cent hypercin, a dose of 250 milligrams St John's wort supplement may be given twice daily. Alternatively, a five per cent hyperforin standardised extracts of the herb may be given at 300 milligrams thrice daily.

Clinical trials on St John's wort have used a wide range of doses, from 0.17 to 2.70 milligrams of hypericin taken orally or about 900 milligrams to 1.80 grams of the supplement daily. Topically, 1.5 per cent of hyperforin has been used for treatment of atopic dermatitis. Children had been given doses of 150 milligrams to 1.80 grams of St John's wort extract daily by mouth which they were able to tolerate.

For other conditions aside from depression, St John's wort may also be given for premenstrual syndrome at a dose of 300 milligrams once daily for standardised 0.3 per cent hypericin extract. For people suffering from other body symptoms of depression, a dose of 300 milligrams standardised hypericin extract is taken every eight hours. Those who are afflicted with somatisation disorder are given a specific commercial extract of St John's wort at a dose of 600 milligrams daily.

Studies on St. John's wort

About 20 million Americans suffering from depression have relied on synthetic antidepressant medications such as fluoxetine and phenelzine. It carries with it side effects such as sleeplessness, headaches, stomach upset, and changes in sexual performance. A 1995 study published in the British Medical Journal suggested that St John's wort is just as effective as the usual antidepressants compared to the placebo in treating mild to moderate depression.

Research has shown that major pharmacologically active ingredients in St John's wort are hypericin, pseudohypericin, and xanthones. However, there are other components in the herb that might contribute to the herb's antidepressant action. Most extract preparations are standardised to 0.3 per cent hypericin at a maximum of 2.7 milligrams of hypericin daily. As with other herbal supplements, the herb can also interact with other medications especially those that affect the immune system.

Several European studies that have shown St John's wort's activity in managing depression are reviewed by the National Institutes of Health (NIH). The experts pointed out the limitations of the study and that there should be rigorous trials to verify the initial data. According to the April 2002 issue of the Journal of the American Medical Association, St John's wort have not been able to prove it is more effective than the placebo on major depressive disorders.

References:

- Your Health Australia. "St. John's Wort: Benefits and Uses of St. John's Wort: Your Health." 2009. http://www.yourhealth.com.au/information-on-natural-medicine-herbs-detail.php?name=St.%20John's%20Wort (accessed 22 Jun 2013).

- Netdoctor. "St John's wort." 2013. http://www.netdoctor.co.uk/diseases/depression/stjohnswort_000316.htm (accessed 22 Jun 2013).

- Patient.co.UK. "St John's Wort." 2010. http://www.patient.co.uk/doctor/St-John's-Wort.htm (accessed 22 Jun 2013).

•   National Center for Complementary and Alternative Medicine (NCCAM). "St. John's Wort | NCCAM." 2005. http://nccam.nih.gov/health/stjohnswort/ataglance.htm (accessed 22 Jun 2013).

My Dr Australia. "St John's wort - myDr.com.au." 2013. http://www.mydr.com.au/mental-health/st-john-s-wort (accessed 22 Jun 2013).

THYME-Thyme is popular culinary herb that is often used as a spice. Its scientific name is Thymus vulgaris and is also referred to common thyme or garden thyme. Other less popular names are French or Spanish thyme and rubbed thyme.

Growing thyme

Being an herb, thyme does not grow any taller than a foot. It's a shrub with small, oval, greyish green leaves. It has tiny tubular, purple or pink flowers that bloom in late spring to summer. It has aromatic woody stems that grow upright.

Thyme has been used initially by the ancient Egyptians for embalming. The ancient Greeks sprinkled it on their baths or smudged it in their temples to inspire courage. The Romans have used the herb for cleansing their rooms and to add flavour to their cheeses and sweetened alcoholic after meal drinks. In the Middle Ages, the Europeans placed packets of thyme under their pillows to induce sleep and deter nightmares.

The kind of thyme currently in used is actually a cultivated form of wild thyme that has been growing in the mountains of southern European countries that border the Mediterranean region. Most countries with temperate climates have cultivated the herb. The short lived herb is propagated with cuttings, seeds, or by dividing the rooted portions of the plant in a warm, sunny location with well-drained soil. It is planted in spring and will tolerate drought well.

Benefits of thyme

As an herb spice, thyme has been a vital ingredient in many dishes. When fresh, recipes will measure thyme in sprigs but when dried, in teaspoonfuls.

Commercial mouthwash and medicated bandages contain thymol, an antiseptic. Infused teas made of thyme are given for people with cough and bronchitis. Thyme is also given for colic, stomach upset, diarrhea, gas, parasitic worms, and stomach aches. Other totally unrelated conditions such as dyspraxia, arthritis, and bedwetting seem to benefit from thyme as well.

Topically, thyme is applied for hoarseness, tonsillitis, sore throat, and bad breath. It has also been rubbed on the scalp for baldness and as an ear drop for the ears to combat fungal and bacterial infections. Thymol is an important ingredient in dental varnish to prevent tooth decay. It may also benefit people with acne.

What to look out for

Very little studies have been done on thyme's safety or possible adverse reaction. However, pharmacokinetic studies on thymol have been able to show that it is cleanly eliminated in the body. It has a mean terminal elimination half-life of 10 hours. Only the sulphate and glucuronide metabolites of thymol have been seen present in urine, but no free thymol is found in the blood or urine.

Common side effects of thyme include headache, lightheadness, low blood pressure, slower heartbeat, irritation of the digestive tract, and muscle weakness. There are some reports of contact dermatitis and allergy when using thyme. People allergic to oregano should be wary of thyme as well. Since thyme can affect blood clotting, people slated for surgery, medical or dental procedure should stop using it at least 14 days before the scheduled procedure. This property of thyme might also potentiate other medications that affect blood clotting such as aspirin, clopidogrel, enoxaparin, warfarin, and other similar drugs.

How to use thyme

Thyme is available dried or fresh. Fresh thyme is flavourful but it might not last a week in storage. Dried thyme retains its flavour and stores better.

Doses with thyme are mostly traditional or label dependent. Most tinctures and essential oils are applied on the skin for fungal infections. Infusions contain five per cent thymol are used as mouthwash and gargles. Diluted thyme oil has been applied in 1 to 2 per cent ointments for many skin disorders.

For people with bald patches, about two to three drops of a mix containing thyme, lavender, rosemary, and cedarwood essential oil set in grapeseed or jojoba is massaged on the bald spots on the scalp every night for as long as seven months. For those with diagnosed paronychia, a drop of 4 per cent thymol in chloroform is applied to the affected area three times daily. When used as a compress for rheumatism, bruises, or other skin disorders, 5 grams of the dried leaves for every 100 millilitres of boiling water is decocted for 10 minutes. It is then strained and soaked in cloth for use as compress.

Children have been able to tolerate thymol when combined in one per cent chlorhexidine as a dental varnish. This mixture has been used every eight hours for 14 days and has shown to prevent periodontal infections from happening.

Studies on thyme

The most valuable medicinal component of thyme is in its essential oil which contains 20 to 54 per cent of thymol. Thymol is a natural antiseptic. The oil may also contain other components such as cymene, myrcene, borneol, rosmarinic acid, and linalool. Other components found from the leaves and aerial plant parts are cadalene, cineole, and terpinene.

A comprehensive study on plants has shown that thymol can be effective against a wide variety of fungi that affect the toenails. According to their data, thymol, carvacrol and cymene have been able to kill species of Candida, Aspergillus, and other fungi. Another separate study by Leeds Metropolitan University has suggested thyme may benefit people with acne.

There are other studies that investigated the activity of thyme's constituents. There are research data that has examined its antioxidant ability. It has also shown some antiplatelet activity in laboratory experiments. Another study has suggested that its ability to inhibit acetylcholinesterase in vitro can be used in managing Alzheimer's disease, although clinical trials have yet to be done.

Animal studies on thyme have been extensive. Thyme extract has shown a relaxant effect on the guinea pig tracheam similar to the bronchdilation caused by theophylline. Another study with mice fed with thyme extracts have been able to demonstrate an increase in an enzyme that will allow glutathione to combine with various free radicals and toxins for ease of excretion from the body.

References:

•   Discovery Fit and Health. "Discovery Health "Thyme: Herbal Remedies"." 2009. http://health.howstuffworks.com/wellness/natural-medicine/herbal-remedies/thyme-herbal-remedies.htm (accessed 22 Jun 2013).

• Nutrition and You. "Thyme herb nutrition facts and health benefits." 2009. http://www.nutrition-and-you.com/thyme-herb.html (accessed 22 Jun 2013).

• Pure Matters. "Thyme." 2011. http://resources.purematters.com/herbs-supplements/t/thyme (accessed 22 Jun 2013).

• RxList. "Thyme Effectiveness, Safety, and Drug Interactions on RxList." 2013. http://www.rxlist.com/thyme/supplements.htm (accessed 22 Jun 2013).

World's Healthiest Foods. "Thyme." 2004. http://www.whfoods.com/genpage.php?tname=foodspice&dbid=77 (accessed 22 Jun 2013).

TURMERIC- Turmeric is a rhizome related to ginger. Its scientific name is Cucurma longa. Other people call it Indian saffron, safran bourbon, or cucurma. Its name is derived from that Latin term "terra merita" meaning merited earth. After processing, it becomes a deep yellow orange powder with a distinct slightly bitter, somewhat hot peppery taste that comes with a smell similar to mustard.

Growing turmeric

The plant can grow up to about five to six feet high and will display dull yellow flowers. It thrived originally in the tropical forests of South and Southeast Asia. The roots are used for food and medicine. Every year, turmeric rhizomes are gathered and grown in the next planting season. Each rhizome has a tough, tan skin that hides its bright orange flesh. These perennial plants need about 20 to 30 degrees centigrade with annual rainfall to reach its full growth potential. At present, India and Pakistan are the major suppliers of turmeric.

Benefits of turmeric

Turmeric has been used initially as a dye for textile before it became a mainstay in Indian Ayurvedic and Chinese medicine. It has been employed as an anti-inflammatory that can treat gas, jaundice, menstrual problems, bloody urine, toothache, bruises, and colic.

The anti-inflammatory activity of turmeric has always been compared with steroids and non-steroidal anti-inflammatory drugs (NSAIDs) minus the side effects (developing ulcers, lowered white blood cell count, or bleeding from the intestines). Being rich in antioxidants, turmeric is said to benefit people who suffer from rheumatoid arthritis. It can neutralise free radicals which when left unchecked, causes pain, inflammation, and gradual damage to the joints.

For affordable treatment for inflammatory bowel disease (IBD) such as ulcerative colitis or Crohn's disease, cucurmin is the key. This substance was able to reduce the usual signs found in IBD induced in mice. At a 0.25 per cent concentration, the effect is visible. It's like eating the same amount of turmeric in curries.

Another major benefit that turmeric can bring is in the field of cancer prevention and development. Cucurmin can destroy mutated cancer cells and prevent them from metastasising in other parts of the body. It does so by improving liver function and preventing a certain protein that provides blood supply to the cancer cell.

Aside from improving liver function, turmeric can also protect the heart and blood vessels. It prevents cholesterol from oxidising. This oxidised cholesterol form plaque that accumulate in the blood vessels. It also directs the genes in liver cells to create more receptors for bad cholesterol. The more receptors binding the bad cholesterol, the faster it is eliminated in the body. Since it is rich in pyridoxine, turmeric prevents homocysteine from accumulating, Homocysteine damages blood vessels directly.

One of the most recent benefits that can be gained from turmeric is its ability to cross the blood-brain barrier which makes it helpful for people who are predisposed to Alzheimer's disease and prevent further deterioration in people with multiple sclerosis. It is believed that it can prevent production of interleukin, a protein that destroys myelin, the protective sheath on the nerves. Its bisdemethoxycucurmin is able to boost the immunity of Alzheimer patients that their amyloid beta plaques are cleared.

What to look out for

As a food, turmeric is very safe. However, when taken as a supplement, try to keep within the recommended doses. Prolonged use of turmeric may cause severe irritation of the digestive tract or worse, develop ulcers. Those with gallstones and problem with their bile ducts should consult with their doctors first before taking in turmeric. It should also not be consumed a fortnight (Two weeks) before surgery as turmeric may exert a blood thinning effect.

Because of such effects, keep an eye out when taking turmeric with medications. It may prevent antacids from being effective. It can also make anti-diabetic medications more potent which could increase the risk of having low blood sugar. Similarly, blood thinning medications (aspirin, clopidogrel, dalteparin, heparin, or diclofenac) can be synergised by turmeric. Herbs such as angelica, cloves, garlic, ginger, gingkgo, ginseng, and willow will also thin the blood when used with turmeric.

How to use turmeric

Southeast Asians incorporate turmeric powder to add color and flavour to their dishes. Indonesians and Indians use turmeric leaves to wrap and cook the food to give the dish its distinct flavour. In the Far East, pickles will contain fresh turmeric made soft by vinegar. Persians cook with it with virtually anything while South Africans add it to boiled rice.

Commercial preparations are sold as capsules, fluid extracts, or tinctures. Bromelain is added to increase its absorption and to boost its anti-inflammatory effects. About 1.5 to 3 grams of freshly cut or dried root may be consumed in divided doses per day. For standardized cucurmin powder in capsules, 400 to 600 milligrams may be given thrice a day. Fluid extracts and tinctures are dissolved in water. For fluid extracts, 30 to 90 drops while tinctures may be 15 to 30 drops every 6 hours daily.

When using turmeric supplements, dosing is important. For dyspepsia, 500 milligrams is taken every six hours. For osteoarthritis and rheumatism, take 500 milligrams every 12 hours.

Fresh turmeric can be kept in the refrigerator. After being picked, turmeric is often boiled for several hours. It is then dried in a hot oven. Once they've cooled down; they are ground to fine powder and kept in a air tight containers in a cool, dark place.

Studies on turmeric

Turmeric's most common active ingredient is cucurmin. This yellow orange pigment has potent anti-inflammatory activity comparable to synthetic medications such as hydrocortisone and ibuprofen.

Most of the recent studies on turmeric are focused on comparing it as an alternative to synthetic drugs. A study in 2008 has shown turmeric being comparable to the effect of atorvastatin. In 2009, a research published how turmeric was able to be 100,000 times more potent than metformin in keeping insulin levels in check. A 2011 study claimed that turmeric has a similar effect to fluoxetine and imipramine in alleviating depression.

References:

•   Medline Plus. "Turmeric." 2012. http://www.nlm.nih.gov/medlineplus/druginfo/natural/662.html (accessed 22 May 2013).

•   Mother Nature Network. "The amazing health benefits of turmeric." 2012. http://www.mnn.com/food/healthy-eating/stories/the-amazing-health-benefits-of-turmeric (accessed 22 May 2013).

- University of Maryland Medical Center. "Turmeric." 2011. http://www.umm.edu/altmed/articles/turmeric-000277.htm (accessed 22 May 2013).

- WebMD. "Turmeric." 2013. http://www.webmd.com/vitamins-and-supplements/lifestyle-guide-11/supplement-guide-turmeric (accessed 22 May 2013).

- World's Healthiest Foods. "Turmeric." 2001. http://www.whfoods.com/genpage.php?tname=foodspice&dbid=78 (accessed 22 May 2013).

UVA URSI- Uva ursi is a small shrub known as a kidney remedy and as an antimicrobial. It is known to many as bearberry and has a scientific name of Arctostaphylos uva-ursi. Other common names are beargrape, hogberry, manzanita, mountain box, rockberry, and sandberry. Bears love eating the edible but sour fruit, hence the name.

Growing uva ursi

Uva ursi is a small shrub that grows close to the ground. It can grow from about two inches to less than a foot high. Its leaves are shiny, smooth and evergreen with lighter undersides. The small, thick, and stiff leaves remain green for about a year or two before falling out. They are arranged alternately on the stems which turn red when planted in full sunlight or green in shaded areas. These stems gradually turn brown and woody as they mature. Pink or white flowers bloom in spring. These urn shaped flowers grow in clusters and eventually bear fleshy fruits. The fruit is a red berry that is smooth and glossy. It grows up to early winter and contains about one to five hard seeds. The seeds have to be scraped thin of their seed coats before they can be sown.

Uva ursi has been used medicinally since the 2nd century. Native Americans have employed it as a remedy for urinary conditions. It has also been employed as an ingredient in Native American smoking blends known as kinnikinnick, where it is mixed with other herbs and tobacco for a narcotic or stimulating effect. Uva ursi is distributed along the Northern Hemisphere and in the mountains of Europe, Asia, and North America.

Benefits of uva ursi

Before the discovery of sulfa drugs and antibiotics, uva ursi has been employed as an antimicrobial for urinary tract infections. Aside from infections, the uva ursi is also given as a mild diuretic, laxative, and for bronchitis. The diuretic effect has made it a natural antihypertensive and a possible herbal alternative for people suffering from congestive heart failure. When combined with other herbs such as hops and peppermint, uva ursi is prescribed for bedwetting. It has also been prescribed with prednisolone and dexamethasone to manage arthritis. Some herbalists have utilised the herb to prevent infection after giving birth, as well as tightening the muscles involved in childbirth.

What to look out for

Uva ursi has hydroquinone, a component that is toxic to the liver. One should never use more than 25 days of uva ursi medication in a year's time. When taken long term, it can cause eye problems such as thinning of the retina, breathing difficulties, convulsions, and death aside from liver problems.

Side effects in using uva ursi are nausea and vomiting, irritability, greenish-brown discolouration of the urine, and sleeplessness. People with certain conditions should not use this herb. Pregnant and nursing women including those suffering from high blood pressure, Crohn's disease, high blood pressure as well as kidney, liver or digestive problems.

Uva ursi supplements can also interact with some medications. Drugs containing lithium and non-steroidal anti-inflammatory drugs, such as ibuprofen or mefenamic acid, might have increased effects when used with uva ursi. Along with the potentiated effects is the increased risk for overdose or side effects. Other supplements such as ascorbic acid and citrus juices might make the urine acidic and diminish uva ursi's effects.

How to use uva ursi

Only the leaves of the uva ursi are used in herbal remedies. Young leaves are often harvested in spring to early summer as they are rich in tannins as well. It is then air dried with exposure to mild heat before being tinctured. Tinctures of uva ursi are given at 2.5 to five millilitres given twice to thrice daily.

Since uva ursi is toxic to children and to some adults, it is best to talk to a healthcare provider before taking it. Most of the doses are dependent on the labelled instructions. The dried herb is often sold in capsules containing 400 to 800 milligrams of arbutin. A maximum dose of two to four grams a day is given. For those who prefer teas, three grams of dried uva ursi leaves are soaked in 150 millilitres of water for 12 hours. It is then strained and served hot or cold every six to eight hours a day. When 15 grams each of uva ursi leaves, poplar bark, and marshmallow root is combined, the mixture is infused in 475 millilitres of water and boiled for 20 minutes. It is then given for kidney stones or inflammation of the urinary bladder. People taking uva ursi orally must also take in a teaspoon of bicarbonate in a glass of water to make the urine alkaline.

Its allantoin content, which has tissue repairing properties, has made the uva ursi leaves as useful for cuts and scrapes including back sprains. The allantoin content has been used in over-the-counter medications for cold sores and vaginal infections.

The use of uva ursi for inflammation of the lower urinary tract has been recognised by the Commission E of the German Federal Institute for Drugs and Medical Devices. Uva ursi should never be used any longer than five days.

Studies on uva ursi

According to research, uva ursi's active components in fighting infections have been due to its arbutin and hydroquinone. Its tannin content, such as gallic and ellagic acid, has the ability to diminish and constrict mucous membranes that helps reduce infections and soreness. Aside from these, it is also rich in flavonoids including hyperoside, myricetin, quercitin in addition to allantoin, coumaric and malic acid. Some studies suggest that the herb works best at the first sign of infection and is more potent when the urine in alkaline; lower pH can destroy its antibacterial effects.

There is data that suggests uva ursi taken with dandelion can reduce the risk of urinary tract infection recurrence in women. However, more studies are under way whether this combination is safe for use long term as uva ursi can damage the liver when taken for some time.

References:

• Ageless. "Information on the herb uva ursi." 2012. http://www.ageless.co.za/herb-uva-ursi.htm (accessed 23 Jun 2013).

• Health Library by iHerb. "Health Library Uva Ursi - Natural, Alternative - 21533." 2010. http://healthlibrary.epnet.com/GetContent.aspx?token=e0498803-7f62-4563-8d47-5fe33da65dd4&chunkiid=21533 (accessed 23 Jun 2013).

• Herb Wisdom. "Uva Ursi Benefits & Information." 2013. http://www.herbwisdom.com/herb-uva-ursi.html (accessed 23 Jun 2013).

• RxList. "Uva Ursi Effectiveness, Safety, and Drug Interactions on RxList." 2013. http://www.rxlist.com/uva_ursi/supplements.htm (accessed 23 Jun 2013).

Your Health Australia. "Uva Ursi: Benefits and Uses of Uva Ursi: Your Health." 2009. http://www.yourhealth.com.au/information-on-natural-medicine-herbs-detail.php?name=Uva%20Ursi (accessed 23 Jun 2013).

VALERIAN- Valerian is a flowering herb that is known for its stinky roots which have calming and sedating effects. Its scientific name is Valeriana officinalis and is also known for its common names all-heal, garden heliotrope, vandal root, capon's tail, and setwall.

Growing valerian

Valerian is indigenous in Europe and some parts of Northern Asia but it has been introduced in North America. It grows along marshy groves and lines ditches and rivers. The plant is often seen conspicuously during summer when their small, fragrant, white or faint purplish pink flowers are in bloom lined with their dark green leaves and set high up the usual vegetation by their tall, hallow stems. The flowers often bloom in late spring. The root is light greyish brown and has a slight aroma when fresh. Dried valerian roots emit a sharp odour.

Benefits of valerian

Valerian is a popular home remedy for insomnia, an alternative herbal remedy from the prescribed sedatives. It has also been given for anxiety and gastrointestinal pain brought about by irritable bowel syndrome (IBS). The relaxing effect it brings about has benefited people suffering from anxiety, agitation, and stress. It has also been taken for lack of concentration, headaches, emotional distress, and spasms caused by menstruation.

Although there isn't enough scientific data to back it up, people with seizures, tremors, attention-deficit hyperactivity disorder (ADHD), hot flashes in post menopause including those with muscle and joint pain have claimed to benefit from valerian use. According to most herbalists, valerian is a versatile nerve tonic and its effect varies on the individual and the situation it is used.

It has been used as an aromatic and diuretic during the time of ancient Greece and Rome. In medieval times, it has been employed as anticonvulsant for different types of epilepsy. Germany's Commission E has recognised valerian for its mild sedative effects. The United States Food and Drug Administration listed valerian as generally recognised as safe (GRAS).

What to look out for

Many people can tolerate valerian because very few side effects have been reported. Drowsiness or dizziness is the most common, especially upon waking up. Large doses of valerian will cause stomach pain, lethargy, mental dullness, or mild depression. Driving or operating heavy machinery or engaging in any activity that requires mental concentration should be performed cautiously or avoided if possible.

Other people have a different reaction to valerian as they might become anxious and restless instead of becoming calm and sleepy. Although valerian does not cause any dependency or any kind of withdrawal symptoms, some people have reported experiencing withdrawal symptoms when taking valerian for very long periods of time. Using valerian any longer than one month must be assessed by a health provider as gradual lowering of the dose is necessary.

Valerian can interact with some medications. The herb can slow down how the liver metabolises certain medications. The drugs can then build up in the body and trigger an overdose. Medications such as antihistamines, some antifungals, and drugs for managing high cholesterol are dependent on liver enzymes in order to be used by the body. Drugs that cause sedation, alcohol, and anaesthetics may have increased effects when used with valerian. The sedative medications can be adjusted by a healthcare providers but those with scheduled surgery or any medical and dental procedures should have their valerian dose lowered at least a month before.

How to use valerian

Valerian supplements are varied in terms of its standardised content of 0.3 to 0.8 per cent valerenic and valeric acids. Other supplements contain ground valerian root. It may also be expressed into fresh juice. It may be sold as capsules, tablets, teas, and tinctures. Commercial preparations combine valerian with sedating herbs including hops, passionflower, skullcap, or lemon balm.

According to the National Institutes of Health (NIH), valerian may be taken at a dose of 400 to 900 milligrams taken at least 30 minutes or two hours before bedtime. Once sleep improves, valerian can be taken for two to six more weeks. Teas can be prepared by steeping a cup of boiling water to two to three grams of dried valerian root in five to 10 minutes. Tinctures are given at four to six millilitres while the fluid extract is taken at a dose of one to two millilitres.

A dose of 200 milligrams of dried powdered valerian extract every six to eight hours daily for anxiety. Alternatively, two cups of valerian tea mixed into a bathtub full of warm water makes for a soothing, relaxing bath. A mix of oils from valerian, nutmeg, and lemon in ammonia is included in the British Pharmacopoeia as a stimulant.

Most products that cater to insomnia contain valerian with other herbs. A product containing 120 milligrams of valerian extract and 80 milligrams of lemon balm extract is given thrice daily for up to a month. Another formulation contains 187 milligrams of valerian extract and 41.90 milligrams of hops per tablet is taken two tablets at a time before bedtime for four weeks.

Studies on valerian

Some of valerian's components have already been identified. It is rich in alkaloids actinidine, chatinine, shyanthine, valerianine, valerenic acid, and valerine including flavanones hesperidin, apigenin, and linarin. It also contains gamma amino butyric acid (GABA), valtrate, and isovaltrate that have been attributed for its medicinal effects. The oil derived from the root appears yellowish green to brownish yellow that is often pungent and earthy like old cheese.

Although the exact mechanism of action of valerian has yet to be determined, scientists hypothesise that valerian increases the amount of GABA in the brain. With GABA in the system, nerve cells are regulated and bring about a calming effect, similar to benzodiazepines such as diazepam.

The herb is a popular safe and gentle alternative for insomniacs. One of the best designed studies on valerian showed that it more effective than placebo in 14 days. After 28 days, the quality of sleep improved significantly which means it might take some time before one can benefit from valerian.

References:

- Ageless. "Information on the herb valerian.." 2012. http://www.ageless.co.za/herb-valerian.htm (accessed 23 Jun 2013).

- American Family Physician. "Valerian - American Family Physician." 2003. http://www.aafp.org/afp/2003/0415/p1755.html (accessed 23 Jun 2013).

- Health Library by iHerb. "Valerian - Natural, Alternative - 21879." 2010. http://healthlibrary.epnet.com/GetContent.aspx?token=e0498803-7f62-4563-8d47-5fe33da65dd4&chunkiid=21879 (accessed 23 Jun 2013).

- Office of Dietary Supplements - National Institutes of Health. "Valerian — Health Professional Fact Sheet." 2013. http://ods.od.nih.gov/factsheets/Valerian-HealthProfessional/ (accessed 23 Jun 2013).

Tang Center for Herbal Medicine Research. "Valerian - University of Chicago." n.d.. http://tangcenter.uchicago.edu/herbal_resources/valerian.shtml (accessed 23 Jun 2013).

WINTERGREEN- Wintergreen is a small shrub which is valued medicinally for its essential oil from its leaves. Its scientific name is Gaultheria procumbens and is also known for its common names such as eastern teaberry, mountain tea, ivory plum, red pollom, chinks, deerberry, wax clusters, or squaw vine. The term wintergreen can also refer to other plants totally unrelated to it. The moxie plum, shallon, pipsissewa, and arctic starflower may also be referred to as wintergreen, as they remain green and lush even through winter.

Growing wintergreen

Wintergreen is a creeping herb native to North America and is related to heath family which includes cranberries, azaleas, and rhododendrons. It is often found on large patches of sandy plains and on mountainous regions. It grows in damp, humus rich soil under the shade. It can withstand low temperatures.

The seeds of wintergreen berries have to be stored at freezing temperatures with moisture for four to ten weeks before it can be sown. The soil has to be enriched with lime-free fertiliser and under shade. The seeds will germinate in one to two months when kept at a temperature of 20'C and enough moisture. It can then be transferred to individual plots after they've reached a height of at least 25 millimetres. It can also be propagated from the roots, which grow from the saplings by late spring or summer. It can be initially planted in clusters and separated after it has developed its own roots.

Wintergreen shrub grows close to the ground at about four to six inches in height. Its evergreen leaves are somewhat oval and is about an inch or two long and about half an inch in breadth and has a characteristic minty fragrance. The shiny leaves are bright green but are pale underneath. It usually appears pale or yellowish green when young and will sport an elliptical shape with slightly jagged edges. As it matures, the leaves become rubbery and lustrous. The stems are stiff and somewhat woody. The drooping, bell-shaped, white flowers bloom from the base of the leaves, usually in late spring. It eventually bears edible berry-like fruit that also carries a minty flavour.

Benefits of wintergreen

Although popular as flavouring, wintergreen has been applied as a topical analgesic and rubefacient in preparations that treat muscle and joint pains. It has also been employed as a diuretic and prescribed for people with chronic discharges in their mucous membrane. It stimulates milk flow and menstruation. The leaves are used for tea or flavouring. As flavouring, it is often mixed with eucalyptus and menthol. The tea relieves flatulence and colic.

What to look out for

Taking large and chronic doses of the oil of wintergreen will irritate the stomach and eventually cause death. Using natural oil of wintergreen might cause skin eruptions and hives because it is easily absorbed by the skin. This which is why many people prefer the synthetic oil of wintergreen, methyl salicylate, or the oil of sweet birch, which are almost identical.

Although generally recognised as safe (GRAS), children should never use wintergreen oil and people with known allergies to any of its components. Those with asthma or any form of gastrointestinal irritation and inflammation should also steer clear of this herb or any of its extracts. Wintergreen oil should not be used longer than three continuous days on a month to month basis.

Wintergreen and methyl salicylate can also potentiate effects of warfarin or any medication that has anticoagulant effect. The oil can also cause poisoning which can be characterised by ringing in the ears, fluid and electrolyte imbalance, and problems in the nervous system.

How to use wintergreen

Since too much wintergreen is lethal, the instruction on manufacturing label should be followed strictly. A dose of wintergreen oil is given at five millilitres which is approximately seven grams of salicylate or about 21.5 adult aspirin tablets. Wintergreen oil is lethal when taken orally.

To make an infusion, boiling water is poured on wintergreen leaves and allowed to steep for a couple of days. The liquid where the leaves have soaked can be heated or cooled when necessary before use. Dried leaves are taken at 500 to 1000 milligrams while the liquid extract of the leaves can be made by one part of the leaves to one part of 25 per cent ethanol and taken at 0.5 to 1.0 millilitres thrice daily. The leaf tea can be gargled for sore throat, douche for leucorrhoea, and as a soaked compress for skin soreness and irritation. A teaspoon of wintergreen leaves can be steeped in a cup of boiling water and drank once daily. The tincture can be taken at a dose of 5 to 15 drops.

Native American Indians have been applying wintergreen leaves directly on skin to treat back pain, rheumatism, fever, headache and sore throat. The edible tart berries were used in pies. The Inuit has eaten the berries raw. The leaves have been used as substitute for tea during the American Revolution and have also been used to relieve colds and muscle aches. It has also been given for nephritis and bladder conditions.

Although the wintergreen leaves can be harvested all year long, the best time is usually in the summer. The leaves are often air dried in the shade before use. Once dry, the leaves are stored in airtight and light protective containers to keep the volatile oil from evaporating. The berries can be gathered during the spring and autumn.

Studies on wintergreen

Initially, the leaves have been recognised by the United States Pharmacopoeia but recently, the oil obtained from the leaves has become official. This volatile oil is often obtained through distillation and comprised of 99 per cent methyl salicylate, with the remaining constituents identified as gaultherilene, salicylic acid and a mix of alcohols, aldehydes or ketones, and esters. Wintergreen oil is not inherent to the plant as it is a product of fermentation between water and gaultherin. To express the oil, the leaves are steeped for 12 to 24 hours before being distilled.

References:

• AltMD. "Wintergreen - Encyclopedia of Alternative Medicine - altMD.com Article." 2008. http://www.altmd.com/Articles/Wintergreen--Encyclopedia-of-Alternative-Medicine (accessed 24 Jun 2013).

• E-Medicine Health. "Wintergreen Effectiveness, How It Works, and Drug Interactions on eMedicineHealth." 2013. http://www.emedicinehealth.com/wintergreen/vitamins-supplements.htm (accessed 24 Jun 2013).

- Georgetown University Medical Center. "URBAN HERBS: Wintergreen." 2010. http://pharmacology.georgetown.edu/urbanherbs/wintergreen.htm (accessed 24 Jun 2013).

- Herbs 2000. "Wintergreen." 2013. http://www.herbs2000.com/herbs/herbs_wintergreen.htm (accessed 24 Jun 2013).

Medicinal Herb Info. "Wintergreen - Medicinal Herb Info." 2010. http://medicinalherbinfo.org/herbs/Wintergreen.html (accessed 24 Jun 2013).

WITCH HAZEL – Witch hazel is a small tree that is highly utilised for its astringent effect. Its scientific name is Hamamelis virginiana and is also known for is common name magician's rod, snapping hazel, spotted alder, tobacco wood, and winter bloom. The term "hamamelis" comes from a Greek word that means similar to the apple tree. It is called witch hazel because it was once the wood of choice for dowsing rods.

Growing witch hazel

Witch hazel is small, woody tree that is indigenous to North America. The leaves are similar to that of the hazel, hence the name.

Witch hazel has a dense mass of stems at its base. Its light brown bark is smooth and the inner bark is reddish purple. The smaller branches often start out smooth and pale brownish orange with dots of white which eventually darken or turn reddish brown. The twigs are flexible and rough with pale green wood. The broad leaves are oval with an oblique base and a rounded apex marked with a wavy toothed margin. The leaves lack any smell but has a bitter aromatic flavour. The leaves drop off in autumn and the flowers appear. The golden yellow flowers have four ribbon-like petals, growing in clusters. It blooms by mid-autumn until the end of autumn. The fruit is hard and woody, almost nutlike, that splits when mature to eject its two shiny black seeds.

Benefits of witch hazel

Witch hazel has been utilised in diarrhoea, tuberculosis, colds, fevers, tumours and some cancers. When applied topically, Witch hazel's astringent effect is beneficial for itching, pain, swelling, varicose veins, haemorrhoids, bruises, insect bites, and mild burns.

Commercial preparations that contain witch hazel are mostly astringent to tighten the skin. Some formulations have been used to decrease or stop bleeding. It may be found in medications for insect bites and stings, teething, haemorrhoids, or itchy, irritated or painful areas of the skin.

What to look out for

Witch hazel is generally safe for most adults when applied directly on the skin. However, there are some people who might experience a slight irritation or stinging. Read the label before using commercial Witch hazel products as some contain isopropyl alcohol which is poisonous if taken internally.

Although most traditional uses for witch hazel might mention using it as tea, taking Witch hazel orally is not recommended because of its high tannin content and the toxicity of the tannin content when consumed has not been scientifically studied. It might be safe when taken in small doses, but there is a tendency to experience stomach upset. Large doses can damage the liver as it has safrole, which is also classified as a carcinogen.

How to use witch hazel

The dried Witch hazel leaves, bark, and twigs are used for herbal remedies. North American Indians have made poultices out of it for painful swellings and lumps. A poultice made of leaves and bark is an effective folk remedy for haemorrhoids as it also alleviates pain. Witch hazel water can be applied up to every two hours or after every bowel movement for itching and discomfort caused by haemorrhoids and similar anal conditions. It is also used for bruises, soreness, and swelling. It may also be made into enemas and suppositories. Ointments and compress made of distilled extracts of the leaves and young leaves of witch hazel are used for varicose veins, insect bites, inflamed eyelids, and bleeding.

Witch hazel's astringent effect makes it effective when taken internally for diarrhoea, dysentery, and mucous discharge. A decoction is given for developing asthma or tuberculosis, inflamed urethra, conjunctivitis, heavy menstruation, and weakness caused by abortion. The tea made from the leaves and bark is good for bleeding and bowel conditions.

Witch hazel may also be used with other herbs. A gargle made from liquid extracts of Witch hazel, myrrh, and cloves can relieve the pain of sore throat or it may be applied to baby's gums during teething. A mouth rinse with witch hazel and myrrh has been used to cure infected gums. A cotton swab soaked in witch hazel, goldenseal, and calendula tea can be plugged in the outer ear to heal swimmer's ear. Tea made with witch hazel, chamomile, mint, and thyme can be taken for stomach flu.

Most of the dosages for witch hazel are mostly based on traditional herbal remedies. A concentrate of fresh leaves is given at two to 11 millilitres. It is then mixed with equal parts of glycerine for haemorrhoids. The liquid extract of witch hazel is made by preparing dried leaves with alcohol and given at six to 18 drops, applied externally for varicose veins and three to six drops for haemorrhoids. Hamamelin, a powdered extract from the bark, is given at 30 to 130 milligrams and when mixed with 65 to 195 milligrams of cacao, makes a good suppository for haemorrhoids. A tincture made from the bark is given as enema, four millilitres of the tincture is mixed with 85 millilitres of cold water as enema for haemorrhoids. Witch hazel lotion is made with 7.5 millilitres of water mixed to 28 millilitres of the extract.

Studies on witch hazel

The tannin content in witch hazel is responsible for its astringent action. The leaves contain tannic and gallic acid, proanthocyanidins, ellagitannins and traces of essential oil that contain safrole and ionon. The bark contains tannin that is partly amorphous and crystalline, gallic acid, phytosterols, resins, fats, and bitter principles. The hamameltannins in the bark also contain catechols.

It also has flavonoids quercentin and kaempferol, saponins, and phenolic acids.

There are scientific data that has shown witch hazel being possibly effective in stopping minor bleeding. Using the bark, leaf or the water on the skin can close up the open capillaries and skin. Its astringent effect has also been found to be useful in relieving itching, irritation, discomfort, and burning caused by haemorrhoids and other similar anal conditions. It is also found to be effective in relieving irritated skin but not as potent as hydrocortisone.

References:

• Ageless. "Information on the herb witch hazel.." 2012. http://www.ageless.co.za/herb-witch-hazel.htm (accessed 24 Jun 2013).

• Herbcyclopedia. "HAMAMELIS VIRGINIANA (Witch Hazel)." 2011. http://www.herbcyclopedia.com/index.php?option=com_zoo&task =item&item_id=77&Itemid=171 (accessed 24 Jun 2013).

• MedicineNet. "WITCH HAZEL (Hamamelis virginiana) - ORAL side effects, medical uses, and drug interactions.." 2013. http://www.medicinenet.com/witch_hazel_hamamelis_virginiana-oral/article.htm (accessed 24 Jun 2013).

• RxList. "Witch Hazel Effectiveness, Safety, and Drug Interactions on RxList." 2013.

http://www.rxlist.com/witch_hazel/supplements.htm (accessed 24 Jun 2013).

University of Michigan Health System. "Witch Hazel | University of Michigan Health System." 2005. http://www.uofmhealth.org/health-library/hn-2186007#hn-2186007-uses (accessed 24 Jun 2013).

YARROW- Yarrow is an astringent flowering herb that is a popular herbal remedy for wounds, cuts, and abrasions. Its scientific name is Achillea millefolium and is also known by other common names such as bloodwort, carpenter's weed, death flower, devil's nettle, field hops, knight's milfoil, stanchweed, old man's pepper, thousand seal, and snake's grass. The term "Achillea" refers to Achilles, a Greek hero who used the plant to heal his wounds while "millefolium" when translated means "coming of a thousand leaves" which pertains to the small, feather-like leaves of the herb.

Growing yarrow

Yarrow is an indigenous plant of the Northern Hemisphere. It is often found in sea level up to elevations of about 11,500 feet. It is commonly found in grasslands and open forests. It also grows in meadows, pastures, and roadsides.

Yarrow has several, upright stems that can grow to about three feet in height. The leaves are distributed throughout the stems in a way similar to a feather, where leaves in the middle are the largest while those on both ends taper down in size in a spiral manner. Each leaf is about two to eight inches, with two or three needle like ends. The flowers are arranged in flattened clusters, about four to nine in a group. Each small flower may be pink or white. The fruits are small, single, and dry similar to sunflowers and dandelions. The whole herb has a strong, sweet scent resembling chrysanthemums and is somewhat hairy with white, silky hairs that lie flat.

Yarrow can grow even in poor soil but it prefers well-drained soil under the full sun. Its flowers bloom from May to June but active growth occurs in spring. Its seeds need light and will germinate when planted no deeper than a quarter of an inch. It needs a temperature of 18 to 24 'C before it can sprout. Its relatively short life can be extended by root division every spring every other year. Its rhizomes can be planted a feet or three apart. It has been cultivated as a companion plant because it repels pests, prevent erosion, and improve soil quality.

Benefits of yarrow

Yarrow is an herbal antibiotic and antispasmodic which makes them an effective home remedy for minor cuts and scrapes. It also promotes excretion of water in form of sweating, salivation, and urination, a helpful property for managing hypertension and relaxing smooth muscles.

Yarrow has been beneficial to people suffering from gastrointestinal conditions such as poor appetite, diarrhoea, dysentery, bloating, gas, and mild stomach cramps. It has also been valuable for fever, common cold, and hay fever. Fresh leaves are chewed for toothache while it has been applied on the skin for haemorrhoids, and wounds. It has also been mixed in soaking baths to relieve painful, pelvic cramps in women and to stimulate menstruation.

What to look out for

People who are allergic to chrysanthemums, daisies, ragweed, and other similar flowers will most probably be hypersensitive to yarrow and its extracts, whether they are taken internally or applied to the skin. Its lactone content might trigger an allergy. The herb can also make the skin more sensitive to ultraviolet light.

Since yarrow can relax the smooth muscles, pregnant women should never take this herb because it might relax the uterus and trigger miscarriage. Animal studies have shown yarrow can also reduce foetal weight and cause sperm abnormality in rats. It should not be used by people with schedule surgery or medical procedure which might involve bleeding.

Yarrow can also interact with certain medications and dietary supplements. It can contradict the effect of blood thinning medications such as aspirin, clopidogrel, warfarin, and other related medications in addition to medications that reduce stomach acids such as cimetidine, esomeprazole, and the like. It can also increase the amount of lithium in the body because of its diuretic effect. Yarrow can also be mildly sedating and medications such as phenytoin, phenobarbital, diazepam, zolpidem, and other related drugs can have an increased effect.

How to use yarrow

Young yarrow leaves are edible and may be consumed cooked or raw. It has a slight bitter flavour that can mix well in salads and as preservative flavouring in beers. Flowers and leaves are made into tea while the oil extracted from the flower heads can flavour soft drinks.

Native American medicine has often included yarrow in its list of herbal remedies. The Navajo have chewed yarrow for toothache and utilised its infusion for earaches. The Miwok, Pawnee, and the Chippewa have employed it as an analgesic and cold remedy. Yarrow tea was drunk by the Cherokee people to cool down fevers and to induce restful sleep. The Iroquois and Mohegan tribes have used it as digestive aid. Traditional Chinese medicine has employed yarrow to affect organs including energy channels. People from the Highlands of Scotland have made it into ointments for wounds.

There is no standard dose for yarrow. Most herbalists rely on the age, health, and other conditions or on traditional doses. Most of the recommended doses are for adults. Yarrow flowers are given as tea or infusion at a total dose of three grams a day. A teaspoon of the dried herb can be added to a cup of boiling water and steeped for 10 minutes. It is then strained and sweetened with honey and taken at bedtime for relaxing sleep. A ratio of 1:1 yarrow extract to 25 per cent ethanol is given at one to four millilitres thrice daily for menstrual bleeding, cramps, or soreness. The dried herb is encapsulated or given as an infusion at two to four grams every eight hours. A ratio of one part yarrow to five parts ethanol tincture is taken at two to four millilitres thrice a day.

Studies on yarrow

Yarrow has pyrrolidine alkaloids betonicine and stachydrine, flavonoids, and volatile principles such as pinene, camphor, cineole, caryophyllene, borneol, camphene, terpinene, limonene, sabinene and azulenic compounds like chamazulene. It also contains salicylic acid which makes it an effective pain reliever and anti-inflammatory.

References:

• Ageless. "Information on the herb yarrow.." 2012. http://www.ageless.co.za/herb-yarrow.htm (accessed 25 Jun 2013).

• Alternative Nature Online Herbal. "Yarrow herb uses, description and pictures." 2007. http://www.altnature.com/gallery/yarrow.htm (accessed 25 Jun 2013).

• Discovery Fit and Health. "Discovery Health "Yarrow: Herbal Remedies"." 2009. http://health.howstuffworks.com/wellness/natural-medicine/herbal-remedies/yarrow-herbal-remedies.htm (accessed 25 Jun 2013).

- Purple Sage UK. "Yarrow." 2005. http://www.purplesage.org.uk/profiles/yarrow.htm (accessed 25 Jun 2013).

Wellness Mama. "Herb Profile: Yarrow-Natural and Herbal Uses." 2009. http://wellnessmama.com/7106/herb-profile-yarrow/ (accessed 25 Jun 2013).

ABOUT THE AUTHOR

Growing up in a family of individuals that valued everything natural Arthur Bramble was actually puzzled by the fact that so many people were seeking the chemically made options from doctors as solutions when everything they needed was right there in nature. He was also bemused by the fact that many of the drugs that are on sale today are extracts of some of the same herbs that they were ignoring.

Not only are herbal remedies safer (when taken in the correct dosages) they tend to have more lasting effects in the long run. He has decided through this book to show that there really is no need to risk some dangerous side effect to get rid of one problem when the herbs are right there to help you alleviate your symptoms in a safer manner. The great thing is that even some doctors today are looking back to herbs as solutions for their patients' problems.

Arthur stands by his work and is a prime example of what herbs can do for the body as he has been using them for years to help with his arthritis and other problems. The book is a must have for every home that is seeking natural solutions to health issues.

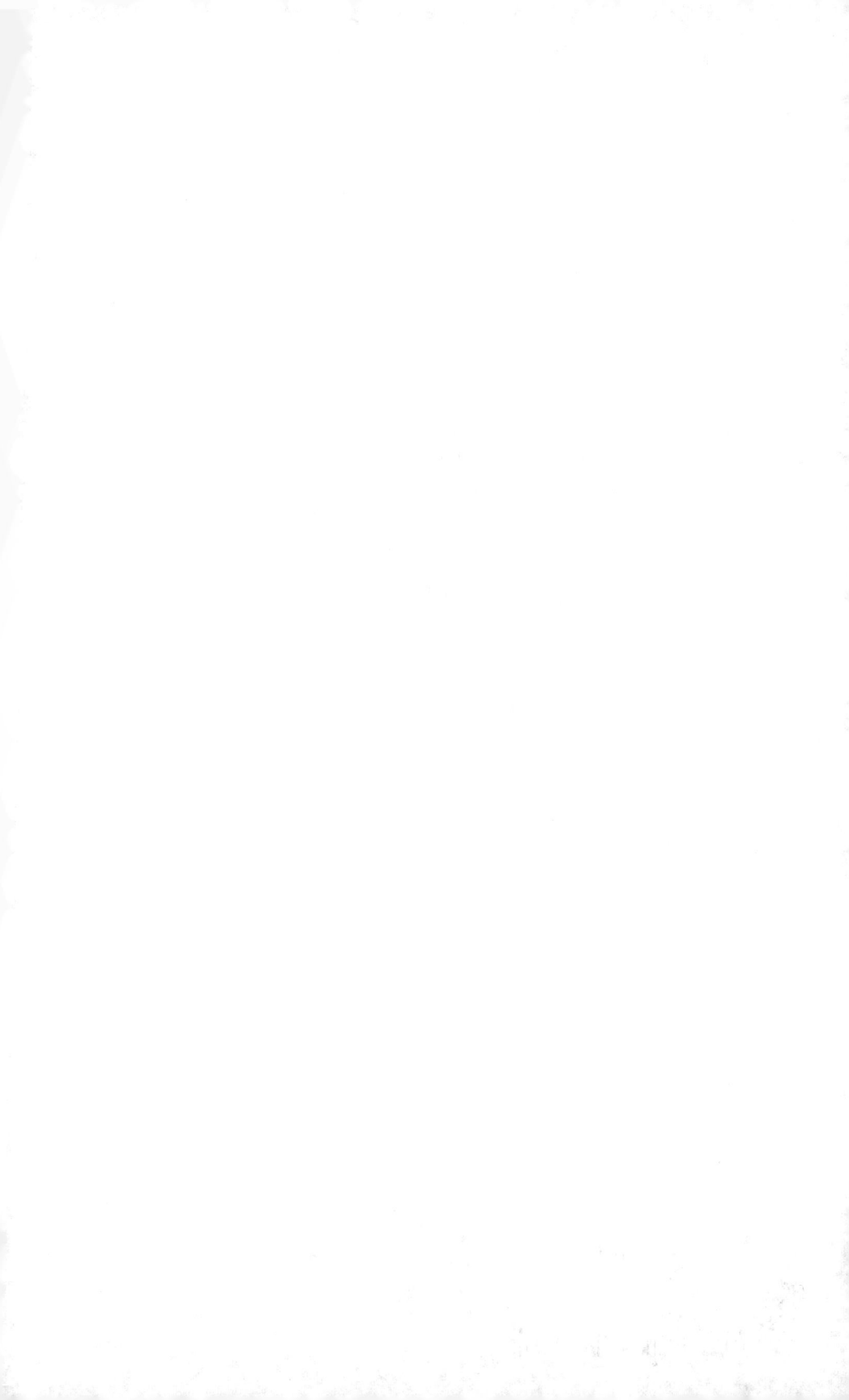

www.ingramcontent.com/pod-product-compliance
Lightning Source LLC
Chambersburg PA
CBHW070627290526
45790CB00001B/23